Chris Stevens began learning the Alexander Technique in 1969. He has been director of a recognized teacher training course for over 10 years and is a former chairman of STAT.

He has carried out scientific research into the Technique in the Department of Anatomy, University of Copenhagen and the Division of Basic Medical Sciences, Kings College, London. Through this, Chris has continued Alexander's tradition using modern scientific methods and advances in scientific knowledge to improve his understanding and teaching methods.

Chris teaches in England and Germany, and has written several books and research papers.

ALEXANDER TECHNIQUE

An introductory guide to the techniques and its benefits

Chris Stevens

Illustrated by
Shaun Williams

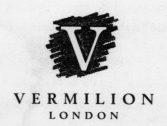

VERMILION
LONDON

First published by Macdonald Optima in 1987

1 3 5 7 9 10 8 6 4 2

Copyright © Chris Stevens 1987, 1995

Chris Stevens has asserted his moral right to be identified as the author of this work in accordance with the Copyright, Design and Patents Act 1988.

This revised edition published in the United Kingdom in 1996
by Vermilion
an imprint of Ebury Press
Random House UK Ltd
Random House
20 Vauxhall Bridge Road
London SW1V 2SA

Random House Australia (Pty) Ltd
20 Alfred Street, Milsons Point, Sydney,
New South Wales 2061, Australia

Random House New Zealand Limited
18 Poland Road, Glenfield,
Auckland 10, New Zealand

Random House, South Africa (Pty) Limited
PO Box 337, Bergvlei, South Africa

Random House UK Limited Reg. No. 954009

A CIP catalogue record for this book is available from the British Library.

ISBN 0 09 180979 7

Printed and bound in Great Britain by Mackays of Chatham, plc

Papers used by Vermilion are natural, recyclable products made from wood grown in sustainable forests.

To my mother

CONTENTS

CONTENTS

ACKNOWLEDGMENTS

With grateful thanks to my colleagues and students, especially Walter Carrington for correcting my many errors.

FOREWORD

This charming little book invites everybody to join in
an exciting adventure. Mostly, we are only too well
aware of our problems in life but we don't realize just
how we could help ourselves. We long for a helping
hand, but we forget to look at the ends of our own
arms.

F M Alexander, whose work this book is about, was
a man with problems; but he was a great explorer, an
explorer of his own capabilities, of his own potential,
of himself. He found a practical way to overcome his
difficulties; and if we follow his example we can re-
discover some of his discoveries and they will prove to
be as exciting for us as they were for him. Since I first
met him, over fifty years ago, and he taught me his
Technique, I have done my best to follow in his tracks
and to help others to do the same; and the further I
go, the more I realize just how far-reaching was his
vision. New vistas of possibility open up all the time.

Chris Stevens has undertaken a similar journey and
he describes some of the views of a new country that
it has opened up for him. He has had a lot of
experience in applying the Technique. He teaches it
professionally and trains students to become teachers,
but he is also involved in a programme of scientific
research to make it more widely known and accepted.
It is not an easy subject to write about because what
it involves is so much a matter of subjective

experience. How can the self-observation of mental and bodily habits, the exploration of our willing and wishing, our thoughts and feelings, be used as a reliable guide for gaining practical ends, still less to establish scientific truth?

The answer is that, if we can bring about evidently beneficial change within ourselves, although the means may be inevitably subjective, the practical results can be evaluated objectively.

To describe such a process to people who have neither had the experience themselves nor observed the results in others must be very difficult. It must involve a long stretch of the imagination. But in this book Chris Stevens has come close to achieving the impossible task. He has not quite managed to square the circle, but he has circled the square and shown us how to get round some of the rough, awkward corners of the problem. The result is a practical, useful, informative book, but above all, with Shaun Williams' amusing drawings, it is enjoyable and much to be recommended.

Walter Carrington, London 1987

INTRODUCTION

The Oscar winning actor, Paul Newman, the conductor, Colin Davis and the authors, Roald Dahl and Edna O'Brien have all spoken of the mental and physical benefits Alexander Technique has brought into their lives. It is also used by Sting to help him relax before a concert, by Barry Tuckwell, the French horn virtuoso, to monitor his body better in performances and by Howard Payne to help him break the Commonwealth hammer throw record. The Alexander Technique has helped thousands of people from all walks of life. Here, in their own words is what some of them have said about it:

Edward Maisel, Director of the American Physical Fitness Research Institute writing on the effects of the Alexander Technique
'There is an overall flexibility and tonic ease of movement, greater freedom in the action of the eyes, less tension in the jaws, more relaxation in the tongue and throat and deeper breathing. There is also a sense of

13

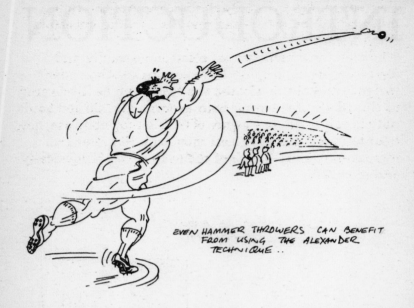

EVEN HAMMER THROWERS CAN BENEFIT FROM USING THE ALEXANDER TECHNIQUE...

weightlessness and a diminution of the effort previously thought necessary to move one's limbs. Activity now becomes free and flowing, no longer jerky and heavy with strain.'

Dr Bent Ostergaard, Consultant Cardiologist, Aarhus University Hospital, Denmark
'The Alexander Technique is a realistic alternative to beta blockers in the control of stress-induced high blood pressure.'

British Medical Journal
'Alexander's work is of first class importance and investigation by the medical profession is imperative.'

Daniel Pevsner, Fellow of the British Horse Society
'The Alexander Technique removed a long standing back problem, improved my riding position and riding ability. Riders who take up the Technique always make a very significant improvement in their riding.'

Professor Raymond Dart, discoverer of the first missing link between man and his ape-like ancestors, *Australopithicus*
'The electronic facilities (of electromyography and electroencephalography) have confirmed Alexander's insights and authenticated the technique he discovered in the 1890s of teaching both average and skilled adult individuals to become aware of their wrong body use, how to eliminate handicaps and thus achieve better (i.e. increasingly skilled) use of themselves, both physically and mentally.'

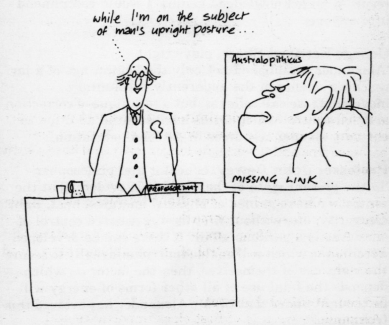

Paul Collins, Canadian National Marathon Champion 1949–52, Veterans' world record holder in 10 events from 200 kilometres to 6 days
'Through the Alexander Technique I was able to rehabilitate my running after 25 years of being unable to run through injuries, to the extent that I was able to set ten world records for veterans in 1982.'

Professor George E. Coghill, anatomist and physiologist
'Mr Alexander's method lays hold of the individual as a whole, as a self-vitalizing agent. He reconditions and re-educates the reflex mechanisms and brings their habits into normal relation with the functioning of the organism as a whole. I regard this method as thoroughly scientific and educationally sound.'

Tony Buzan, inventor of Mind Maps, author of *Use Your Head* and *The Evolving Brain*.
'The Alexander Technique transformed my life. It is the result of an acknowledged genius. I would recommend it to anyone.'

George Bernard Shaw, playwright
'Alexander established not only the beginnings of a far reaching science of the apparently involuntary movements we call reflexes, but a technique of correction and self-control which forms a substantial addition to our very slender resources in personal education.'

Professor John Dewey, educator and philosopher
'In the present state of the world it is evident that the control we have gained of physical energies, heat, light, electricity, etc, without first having secured control of ourselves is a perilous affair. If there can be developed a technique which will enable individuals really to secure the right use of themselves, then the factor on which depends the final use of all other forms of energy will be brought under control. Mr Alexander has evolved this technique.'

Sir Charles Sherrington, Nobel prizewinner for physiology and medicine
'Mr Alexander has done a service to the subject by insistently treating each act as involving the whole integrated individual, the whole psychophysical man. To take a step is an affair not of this or that limb solely

but of the total neuromuscular activity of the moment
– not least of the head and neck.'

John Cleese, comedian and actor
'I find the Alexander Technique very helpful in my work.
Things happen without you trying. They get to be light
and relaxed. You must get an Alexander teacher to show
it to you.'

Aldous Huxley, writing of the Alexander Technique
'It is now possible to conceive of a totally new type of
education affecting the entire range of human activity,
from the physiological, through the intellectual, moral
and practical, to the spiritual – an education which, by
teaching them the proper use of the self, would preserve
children and adults from most of the diseases and evil
habits that now afflict them.'

W H M Carrington, writing on the Alexander
Technique
'Our human upright posture is a unique accomplishment
. . . a most delicate balance, an equation of forces brought
about by an interplay of the sensory and motor
mechanisms, by which all muscular effort is practically
eliminated. The unique quality of the whole performance
lies in this reduction of effort.'

Professor Frank Pierce Jones, author of *Body
Awareness in Action: A Study of the Alexander
Technique*
'The Alexander Technique doesn't teach you something
to do. It teaches you how to bring more practical
intelligence into what you are already doing; how to
eliminate stereotyped responses; how to deal with habit
and change. It leaves you free to choose your own goal
but gives you a better use of yourself while you work
toward it . . . It opens a window onto the little known
area between stimulus and response and gives you the
self-knowledge you need in order to change the pattern

of your response – or, if you choose, not to make it at all.'

F M Alexander
'Every man, woman and child holds the possibility of physical perfection; it rests with each of us to attain it by personal understanding and effort.'

In this book I aim to explain why so many people have found the Alexander Technique helpful. In addition I want to communicate something of the process Alexander went through, not just because of historical interest, but because to learn the Technique each of us has to undertake a similar journey. Although a map is no substitute for real countryside, even a rough sketch map helps us to find our way in unknown terrain. I hope this guide will give you some views of a new country.

1.
WHAT IS ALEXANDER TECHNIQUE?

In 1894 a young Australian actor began to teach a method for improving the way we use our bodies. His name was Frederick Matthias Alexander and his technique was soon being used by fellow actors. Later singers, dancers and musicians began to use it to improve their performance (today it is taught in leading drama and music colleges).

Some of his amateur colleagues were doctors and it quickly became obvious to them that, although the Technique was not a therapy, it did have therapeutic effects. These physicians, having tested the Technique on themselves, began sending some of their patients to Alexander. The first of these were people with breathing problems; since then the Technique has proved useful in a wide range of complaints.

As Dr Wilfred Barlow, a leading consultant in physical medicine at a London hospital reports, the Technqiue can also be used beneficially in stress-related diseases such as ulcers and other digestive disorders, some forms of heart disease and high blood pressure, asthma and chronic bronchitis, tension-related sexual disorders, epilepsy and migraine. He found it of particular use in the rehabilitation phase of many illnesses. The range of rheumatic disorders from disc lesions, low back pain, arthritis, to tennis elbow and frozen shoulders also respond well. In the area of mental health, Barlow reports that the Technique has had considerable success in helping patients suffering from anxiety and depression.

This combination of improvement of performance and better health was well summarized by Nobel Prizewinner for Medicine and Physiology, Professor Nikolaas Tinbergen in his acceptance speech, when he reported '. . .very striking improvements in such diverse things as high blood pressure, breathing, depth of sleep, overall cheerfulness and mental alertness, resilience against outside pressures, and also in such a refined skill as playing a stringed musical instrument'.

Alexander moved from Australia to London in 1904 with letters of introduction from a leading Australian surgeon to his colleagues in London. Some of the latter recognized the usefulness of his Technique and co-operated with Alexander until his death in 1955. This support continues today as we will see in more detail later.

ALEXANDER AND HIS DISCOVERY

Alexander was born in 1869 on the island of Tasmania. He grew up in the country and, although he started at the local school, bad health made it impossible for him to continue, and he was taught at home. Alexander developed a passion for Shakespeare and at an early age resolved to become an actor. He developed a repertoire of humorous monologues and Shakespearean speeches.

Throughout his early life, FM, as he was later to be called, suffered from poor health. He had been born prematurely and only survived due to his mother's ingenuity and persistence in finding a way to feed her

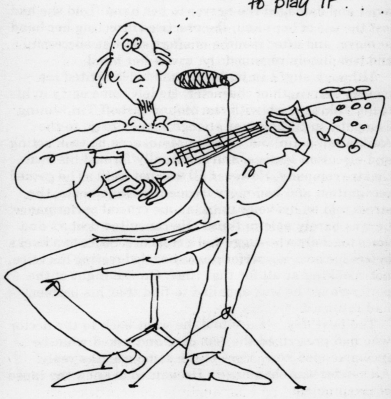

This next piece is dedicated to F.M. Alexander, without whom I would not be able to play it . . .

infant. His mother was a remarkable woman, who acted as the local midwife. Alexander told how he remembered that often, when responding to an urgent call, she would jump her horse over the farm fence, rather than wait to open the gate. Later, when FM was in London, she travelled from Australia to stay with him. One day, whilst crossing a road, she fell and her hand was run over by the wheel of a horse-drawn delivery van. This broke her wrist and damaged the nerves to her hand. Told she had lost the use of her hand, she practised directing her hand to move, and after months of effort she was successful and completely regained the use of her hand.

Although slight in build, Alexander inherited his mother's strength of character. He left home early in his teens, taking a job with the Mount Bishoff Tin Mining Company until he saved enough money to go to the Australian mainland. Once in Melbourne he took acting and elocution lessons, and eventually formed his own theatre company. However all was not well; as he gained recognition and had more frequent engagements, the stress told on his voice until, at one crucial performance, he was barely able to finish. He consulted doctors and voice teachers who suggested a rest cure. So for two weeks before his next big performance he tried resting his voice, not speaking at all for that time. On the night of the performance he was appalled to find that his problem had returned.

The next day, we are told, he went back to the doctor who had prescribed the rest cure and asked what he recommended now. More of the same was the reply. Alexander was not amused. He wanted to know the cause of the problem.

'Is it not fair, then,' he asked, 'to conclude that it was something I was doing that evening in using my voice that was the cause of the trouble?'

'Yes, that must be so,' replied the doctor.

'Can you tell me, then,' asked FM, 'what it was that I did that caused the trouble?' The doctor admitted that he could not.

'Very well,' said Alexander, 'if that is so, I must try and find out for myself.'

However this was easier said than done. He did have some clues to go on: firstly, he knew that the problem had something to do with what he did on stage as he did not have problems with his voice when he was not acting; secondly, his friends told him that when he was on stage he made a loud gasping sound as he breathed in between lines — you can hear this often today with singers, actors and public speakers, particularly when they are nervous.

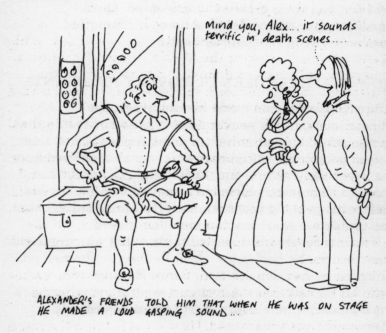

ALEXANDER'S FRIENDS TOLD HIM THAT WHEN HE WAS ON STAGE HE MADE A LOUD GASPING SOUND ...

Alexander decided to observe himself in a mirror, first when he spoke normally and then when he recited to see if he could detect any difference. He began to notice a pattern emerging. When he got ready to recite he drew in air with a noisy gasp, at about the same time he tensed his neck muscles which pulled his head back and down. He also found that this made him compress his vocal cords. Finally he noticed that he had made his whole body shorter and tenser, restricting his breathing and general freedom of movement. When he looked again at his normal speaking, he found the same tendencies, just less so.

By means of careful experiment Alexander found a way of preventing the pattern from starting. He did this by not allowing himself to 'get ready' in his habitual way. He then made use of his observations to find new and better ways of using the various parts of his body involved in reciting. The result was, that after a long period of practice, his voice problem disappeared. Quite unexpectedly, Alexander also noted a dramatic improvement in his general health.

HOW IS ALEXANDER'S DISCOVERY RELEVANT?

After Alexander had made his discovery, the improvement in his performance was so noticeable that people asked him what he had done. As he showed them, it soon became clear that many of them also suffered from the same general problem. Originally Alexander had thought that the problem only applied to him, but his observations and discussions soon led him to believe that the problem was a very common one indeed.

To show people what he meant about the way they held their bodies, he had to get them to observe themselves, much as he had done in the mirror. Because this was difficult (it had taken Alexander several years to make his discovery), he quickly learnt to guide people's movements with his hands.

Today most teachers of the Alexander Technique use the same method. Starting with simple actions, such as sitting, standing, walking and lying down, the teacher and student work together to pinpoint the ways in which the student habitually uses his body incorrectly.

With the practical help of the teacher the student can learn how to stop such harmful habits. This is usually done through a combination of demonstration, verbal

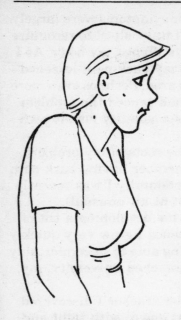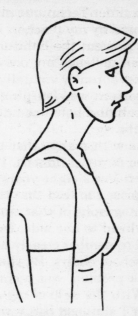

PUTTING THE HEAD BACK
AND DOWN AND SHORTENING
THE BODY WHEN UNDER STRESS.

THE RESULT OF
'GIVING DIRECTIONS'.

instructions and gentle guidance with the hands. The latter is especially important to give the student a reliable experience of what it actually feels like to use his body correctly. As a result the student learns how to let the body work in a freer and more natural way. Once this has become established it is possible to apply the principles to more complex and demanding situations.

As they progress students often realize how their specific problems or symptoms were caused by the general misuse of their bodies. My own experience may make this clearer.

I first took Alexander lessons because of persistent back pain. I had tried conventional medical treatment, osteopathy and yoga. All gave short-term relief but the pain kept coming back. When I went for lessons in the

Alexander Technique my specific symptoms were largely ignored by my teacher. Instead I was helped to recognize and prevent the habitual way I stiffened my body. As I began to 'leave my body alone', my back pain lessened and eventually virtually disappeared. Perhaps even more important was learning how I had caused the problem myself and how I could take responsibility for my own wellbeing.

As with many other things the roots of my problem were in my childhood. I can remember having back pain when I was eight years old (incidentally I was recently surprised to find that this is not at all unusual). Photographs of that time show me developing a tilt of my head to one side. In adolescence I grew very quickly and remember clearly never being able to sit comfortably in school chairs. By the time I reached university, my back problem was a chronic one.

With the help of my Alexander teacher I discovered that I slumped badly when I sat down, with tight and short belly muscles pulling down on my ribs and spine, forcing my head and shoulders forward, which in turn caused my neck, shoulder and back muscles to be under considerable strain. I learnt gradually how to let go of the shortening of the belly muscles by directing them to release, a sensation my teacher was able to help me actually experience through the skilful use of his hands. The result – I slumped less and my breathing was easier because the ribs could move more freely; my head balance improved as he helped me to release the excessive tension and shortness in my neck muscles; similarly, my shoulders, which had always been very rounded, began to broaden and take up a naturally straighter position; and I gained an inch in height and broadened around my chest as well as my shoulders – to the extent that after a while my shirts and jackets became too small for me.

My own experience underlines the fact that the Alexander Technique is not a therapy. Instead I was learning how to allow my whole body to work in an

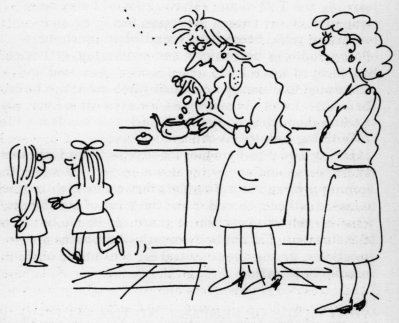

I like to put aside a little each week for therapy when they grow up...

AS WITH MANY OTHER THINGS THE ROOTS OF THE PROBLEM WERE IN CHILDHOOD...

unrestricted, more natural way. In my case, certain symptoms were cleared up as I learnt the Technique, but such 'cures' are incidental and the usefulness of the Technique is in no way dependent on them. (In fact, as I have learnt in my research, there are many causes of back pain that are not related to body use, and any prospective student who suffers from back pain should be aware of this fact.) However, as I discovered for myself, there are other, even more important, reasons for learning the Technique. Firstly, I found I was more competent in my chosen activities, lecturing and practising yoga. Secondly, I found I had much more energy and took up running and swimming, activities I had dropped when I left school, and was excited and stimulated to discover I could do these activities better than when I was a teenager. At the same time I was able to think more clearly and went back into academic life, researching into the Technique.

Having said this, I am pleased to report that I still have my problems and am by no means perfect. However the Technique has given me a set of practical tools with which to tackle difficulties and make the most of my talents. What is even more exciting is there appears to be no end to the process. Each new discovery illuminates a new possibility, giving the potential for continuing and self-sustaining growth.

WHAT KINDS OF PEOPLE FIND THE TECHNIQUE USEFUL?

Jane H is a pianist of many years experience. She had had a successful concert career and taught in a conservatoire. However, she confided to me, she had a problem with her playing. A particular piece required a long and fast arm movement to reach a high note. She had spent a great deal of time trying to improve her technique, but the sound of the note remained unsatisfactory.

She demonstrated the piece for me and it soon became clear that before she began to move her arm she was tightening her neck and hunching her shoulders just enough to affect the movement but not enough to be noticed by the casual observer. I was able to alert Jane to this muscle tensing and show her how to stop it happening. As she progressed Jane found that her ease of playing and the quality of the note improved. An additional bonus was her increased enjoyment of playing.

Jane's example illustrates how the Technique can improve performance. So often skilled performers, be they in sport, music, acting, or whatever, have seemingly unimportant habits of body use that actually undermine their chances of success. It is not usually possible to correct such problems immediately; a course of basic lessons that deals with the person's whole body is needed first, then once the Technique has been mastered, it can be applied to improving a particular skill.

Mr G is a dentist, who came to me complaining of neck and shoulder pain. When we first met the muscles of his neck and shoulders were indeed tight, but so were those of his belly, back, arms and legs. We worked together to unravel what was cause and what was effect.

From this it became clear that the pains were caused by Mr G literally pulling himself out of shape in his work, mainly by an overcontraction of his chest and belly muscles and poking his head forwards. Once he realized he was doing this and was taught how to prevent it, the pains began to abate.

This kind of problem is common. For a variety of reasons people develop habits of body use which produce so much stress in the body that painful symptoms result. Finally it is important to notice that we did not attempt to treat the symptoms directly. Instead, we found the cause of the body misuse that underlay them.

Don't worry — this injection isn't for you..

MR G IS A DENTIST — HE SUFFERED FROM NECK AND SHOULDER PAIN.....

Elizabeth K is a respected psychotherapist. Some of her colleagues had told her about the Alexander Technique and she decided that, although she had no specific problems, she would like to know how to use her body in a more natural way. When we began working together it was obvious that she was a very intelligent and sensitive person. She quickly felt the freedom and lightness in her body increasing. More interesting for her was the experience of the connection between thoughts, feelings, and the way the body works. She was already aware of the existence of this link from her own work with the emotions, but the closeness of the connection was a revelation to her. She was particularly fascinated by the direct link between thought, the aliveness of the body and positive emotional changes.

Elizabeth is an example of a growing number of people who take lessons in the Alexander Technique, not because of health or performance problems, but because they find it a valuable tool for improving their wellbeing and self-knowledge.

2.
WHY WE NEED ALEXANDER TECHNIQUE

BODY MISUSE AND MODERN LIVING

'We live in a time of rapid change' is a phrase in constant use these days. Usually, it is used to refer to technological advances, scientific breakthroughs and so on, but it also applies to us as a society – ideas change, different political parties come and go, social norms shift (note, for example, the recent upsurge in divorce). Obviously we as individuals are affected too. What do such upheavals do to our bodies, not to mention our minds and relationships? In simpler, more stable societies the body use of ordinary, healthy people is quite different from those we see in contemporary westerners. In the process of making his discovery Alexander began to think about the causes for this.

He suggested that under natural conditions only the creatures with good body use survive, those who are clumsy and slow perish. Under these relatively unchanging conditions successful creatures naturally tend to have good body use. But with the rise of agriculture and the growth of cities a great change occurred. The body was less and less used in a spontaneous and natural way. It was more and more restricted to a narrow range of activities. At the mental level, thought became ever more complex and the increase of formal education accentuated this.

In short there has been a rapid and increasing change in the demands on human beings which has caused a general change in the way humans operate. They have become less and less physical, more and more mental, more and more static, and more and more complicated. It has led one critic of civilization to call modern humans 'homo-sedens' – the 'sitting human'.

It must be remembered that human evolution has taken at least five million years, only the last 10,000 of which can be said to have been civilized. This would imply that our biology is 99.9 per cent based on the relatively unchanging demands of nature. Only a very small percentage has had time to adapt to the new and rapidly changing conditions of civilization.

Before modern time, the slow rate of change allowed humans to gradually and unconsciously adapt the body to new conditions. Now, however, it is we who change the environment, and we do it more and more rapidly. Think for a moment of your day, from when you wake up in the morning, and contrast it with what living in the wild must have been like: sleeping in a soft bed; being woken up by a sudden mechanical or electronic noise; the almost instantaneous change from dark to light as we switch on the bedside light in winter; sitting, in a chair at breakfast, in a bus or train or car, at work, after work; walking down a street on a hard pavement, often within a few feet of fast moving and noisy vehicles, each of which can be bigger, faster and noisier than any animal; reacting to events we cannot hear or see directly via telephone, radio and TV Is it any wonder many of us become over-tense and collapse in a heap at the end of such a day?

Proprioception

The changes mentioned above are only a few of those that occur constantly in our everyday lives. In total they are more dramatic and wide ranging than we imagine. As a result of this tension in our bodies, the information our brains receive about where parts of the body are and what they are doing relative to each other, whether they are moving or still, is less reliable than when we lived in the wild. This information concerning the state of the body is called proprioception, and comes mainly from the joints, tendons and muscles. The importance of proprioception can hardly be exaggerated. It is the basis for balance, posture and movement. Even more fundamental, it is the basis for our sense of self. This aspect of proprioception is vividly illustrated by the neurologist Oliver Sacks, who reported one of his case studies about a woman who lost almost all proprioception. Her accompanying loss of her sense of self and her emotional, as well as physical, difficulties make harrowing reading.

Re-educating our proprioception

What we have not done, Alexander suggests, is to apply our reasoning to how we can learn to react in a better way to these changed circumstances and re-educate our proprioception so that it becomes reliable once more. We have not noticed the general deterioration in the way we use our bodies due to our loss of proprioceptive acuity. We do not consider the possible effect of the general misuse of our bodies on our ability to carry out both every-day and skilled actions, on our health and even on our underlying psychological state. Instead we only notice specific symptoms and then try to treat them in isolation. We do not see, for example, that our headache is connected to the way we are using our whole body.

Alexander was not suggesting that all our problems are caused by misuse of the body, but that it can be a factor which in many instances is the dominant one.

Moreover, almost all of us misuse our bodies to some extent, which has to affect us adversely in a variety of ways.

Diana K is a dancer. After a successful professional career, she began to question her work. This led her to explore various styles of dance and other disciplines including the Alexander Technique. In the course of her lessons she found that she was holding her body in a rather fixed and rigid way, especially when she began to dance. Although she was very flexible, the amount of movement she could coax from her body actually came from forcing it to move, and, as with many other dancers, this had led to nagging injury problems. As we worked she found that she could approach her dance in a more relaxed, natural way, opening up new creative opportunities for her dance and incidentally reducing her injury problems.

HOW MISUSE MANIFESTS ITSELF

When a number of scientists looked closely at the way most people stand, they came up with surprisingly similar results, results which did, in fact, differ quite markedly from the pictures we see in anatomy textbooks (see diagram A on page 38).

In most people the head and the pelvis are in front of the body (see diagram B on page 39). The curves of the neck and upper back are exaggerated and there is a flattening of the curve in the lower spine. Notice how the balance of the body is in front of the ankle joints.

In dancers we often see a different pattern (see diagram C on page 39). Here the neck and upper back are over straight and the lower back has a large curve, with the legs being stiff and straight. In such cases the balance of the body is further back, but the body is rather tense.

With students of the Alexander Technique the body tends to look more like that in diagram A, but in a free and natural way and with great individual variations. It must be emphasized that these changes, and others detailed later, are not the result of simply trying to stand up straight. They come about naturally when the body is allowed to use the proper mechanisms.

HOW ALEXANDER STOPPED MISUSING HIS BODY

The short answer to this question is by stopping pulling his head back and down and making himself shorter and narrower. Although this is factually correct, it does not tell us *how* he did it. And without the practical experience it is difficult to explain.

However the discoveries Alexander made can be described fairly simply. Studies have shown how we pull ourselves out of shape. The curves in the spine, for instance, are usually distorted, the ribs narrowed and the balance of the head disturbed, usually as the result of muscles contracting and shortening too much.

'Primary control'

The first step to preventing distortion of the spinal curves and other parts of the body happening, Alexander discovered, was to refuse to act immediately. The next step was to achieve lengthening of the muscles by 'directing the head forward and up without stiffening and narrowing the back. Alexander called this skill 'a primary control', primary because it is the first action that must be working correctly if proprioception and other senses are to be improved. This in turn allows improvements in balance, posture and movement – three key factors affecting health and performance. Refusing to act too hastily allows muscles to decontract, while operating the primary control allows muscles to lengthen by the mechanisms described below.

As we shall see later there is good reason to believe that the improvement in balance reduces muscle tension and the chance of damage to muscles and bones. Improved

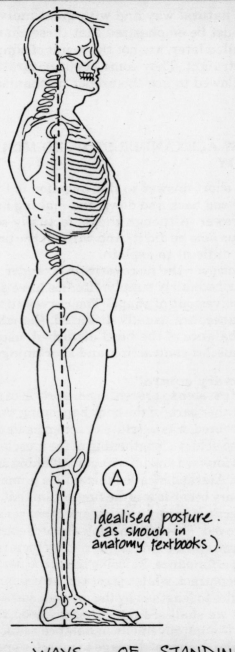

(A)

Idealised posture.
(as shown in
anatomy textbooks).

WAYS OF STANDING.

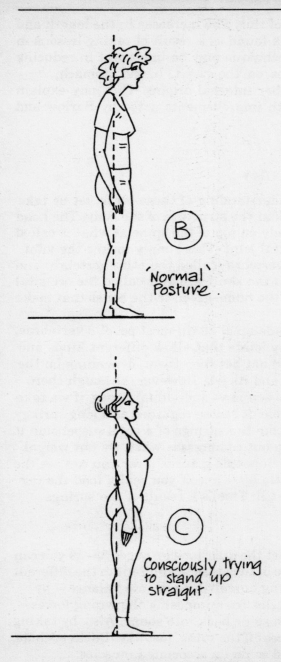

B

'Normal' Posture.

C

Consciously trying to stand up straight.

posture is a part of this. The increases in the length and width of the trunk found as a result of taking lessons in the Alexander Technique may be important in reducing harmful pressures on the heart, lungs, stomach, intestines and other internal organs. This may explain some of the health improvements noted by Barlow and Tinbergen.

A LITTLE ANATOMY

To help in the understanding of these ideas, let us take a very simple look at the structure of the body. The head balances very freely on top of the spine at what is called the atlanto-occipital joint. This simply means the joint between the top vertebra (called the atlas-vertebra) and the bottom part of the skull which is called the occipital bone (vertebra is the name given to the bones that make up the spine).

The spine is made up of 33 (in most people) vertebrae, linked together by joints that allow different kinds and amounts of movement between them, depending on the part of the spine and its job. However, although there is movement between most individual bones, if we take the spine as a whole, it can be regarded as a long springy curved column. Like the springs of a car's suspension it holds the body up but compresses when we put weight on it – just as when people get into a car you can see the car go down a little bit – and if you really load the car up it gets lower still. This is a result of the springs bending.

'Lengthening'
If you look again at the diagrams on pages 38–39 you can see that the shape of the spine is different in the different diagrams. Bringing ourselves back into balance – by stopping the muscles from imposing the wrong forces – tends to bring the spine back into shape. Also, by taking the excessive forces off the spine, just like the car springs, it gets longer and so do its associated muscles.

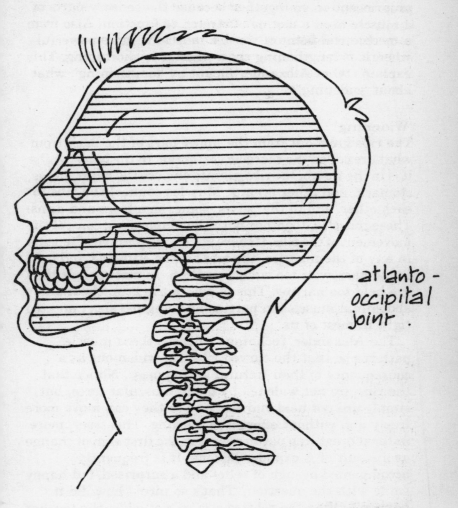

atlanto-
occipital
joint.

THE HEAD AND NECK VERTEBRAE

The lengthening of a muscle and improvements in proprioception go together because the sensory parts of a muscle need a degree of stretch to function. Also from a mechanical point of view, a muscle is more powerful when it is lengthening than when it is shortening. This explains what Alexander meant by 'lengthening', what about 'widening'?

'Widening'

The ribs grow out from the upper part of the back from what are called the thoracic vertebrae. In the baby, whilst it is in the womb, the ribs grow to enclose the heart, lungs, stomach, and other organs. Muscles connect the ribs to each other, and to the pelvis, spine, shoulders and arms. These muscles, together with the diaphragm, control the movement of the ribs. If there is a wrong pattern of tension in any of the muscles, the ribs can be stiffened and held in too narrow or too wide a position. In most people they are held too narrow. This is due to the arm, chest and abdominal muscles in particular being too short and too tight in most of us.

The Alexander Technique releases these muscle patterns so that the curved ribs can widen out as a consequence of their natural springyness. Notice that the ribs are not widened by using muscular force, but simply are not held 'narrow' and so they can move more freely and without effortful breathing. This freer, more natural breathing pattern is often the first sign of change as a result of Alexander lessons. It is frequently accompanied by sigh of relief and a surprised, but happy smile with the question, 'That's so nice – how did it happen?' Often the release occurs, not when the teacher is working on the abdomen or chest as one might expect, but when their hands are on the neck. From very early on Alexander found that the neck was a key part of the primary control. He was not an anatomist and did not concern himself with being more precise than just talking about the neck. Later, when physicians and scientists first tried to understand why the Alexander

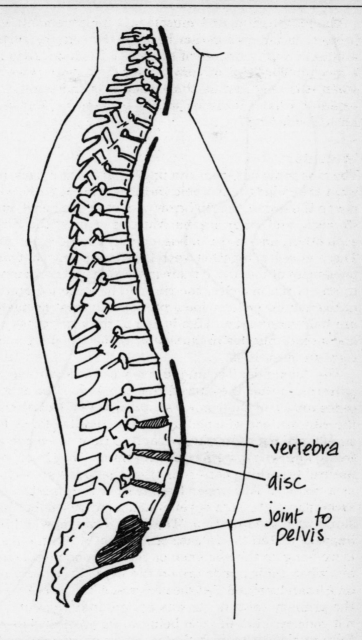

vertebra

disc

joint to pelvis

THE CURVES OF THE SPINE

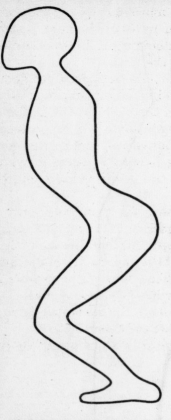

HEAD RETRACTION
IN SITTING DOWN

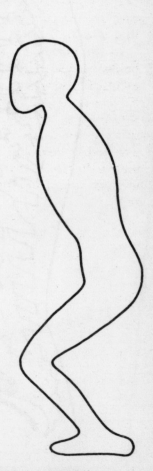

BETTER BODY USE IN
SITTING DOWN

Technique was effective in a more exact way, they were tempted to look for particular parts of the neck — some voted for the muscles just outside the atlanto-occipital joint, others for the joints in the neck.

Alexander himself, however, did not speculate about which parts of the neck were important, but focused on the practical point that when the neck is stiff and short it pulls the head down, causing in some way, a shortening and narrowing of the body. Conversely, when the neck is allowed to release, and the head is directed forward and up, the trunk as a whole can be directed to lengthen and widen.

Alexander did not think of the primary control as only being to do with the head and neck. In fact he found that much of his problem was to do with his interference with his legs and feet. He also taught the importance of the fact that the way we use our arms affects the body as a whole. In short we have to be concerned with the whole of our psycho-physical self. The head–neck relationship is by no means the whole story; it is rather to be seen as an important *indicator* of the use we are making of our whole self.

3.
HOW ALEXANDER TECHNIQUE HELPS

Having seen the detrimental effects of poor posture and misuse of the body generally, the question now is how can we go about learning to stop interfering with the balance of the body?

To find some answers to this question we need to go back to Alexander's own experience for, as you may already have guessed, learning the Technique is not just a matter of knowing what should happen and making it happen. If you have any doubts about this, try demonstrating to an Alexander teacher what you think you have learned so far from this book.

THREE FUNDAMENTAL DISCOVERIES

In some ways you are roughly at the point where Alexander was when he had made his original discoveries. However, when he first tried to apply his findings to himself during his public recitations, he found he slipped back to his old habits almost immediately. So Alexander had to start again. By very careful observation

47

of exactly what he did, he was led to three further
fundamental discoveries.

'End gaining' and the 'means whereby'

First, that the habits he was dealing with were far more
deep-rooted and powerful than he had at first thought.
The most serious of these, he found, was the tendency
to try to act immediately. The best analogy for this is
walking across a busy road: if we just 'do it', we are liable
to be run over; instead we have to stand at the kerbside,
look and wait until there is no traffic and it is safe. This
is an action we have to learn consciously and by repetition
– no doubt you remember being taught your 'kerb drill'
as a child. In the end the routine is almost automatic
(we will return to the importance of the 'almost' later).
This habit of going directly for things Alexander called
'end gaining'. Its opposite, the process of waiting,
observing and working out what must and must not
happen so we can perform the action safely and well he
called attending to the 'means whereby'. (Incidentally
it was learning these concepts from Alexander that led
Aldous Huxley to write his book *Ends and Means*.)

'Faulty sensory appreciation'

His second important realization was that these habits
were not just habits of action, but that, like the habit
of running our fingers through our hair, there were habits
of feeling (proprioception) underlying the habitual
actions. It was the habitual, unnoticed feelings from his
body that he was relying on to do the action. So much
so that, if he did prevent his habitual stiffening and
tightening before an action, it felt quite wrong to him.
This shows just how fundamental proprioception is and
how central proprioceptive habits are to the way we use
our bodies.

It is quite common for students, when they have been
helped to release their body, to feel twisted or that they
are leaning backwards or forwards, when in fact they
are now straight and vertical for the first time. As you
can guess this sets up a vicious circle preventing change.

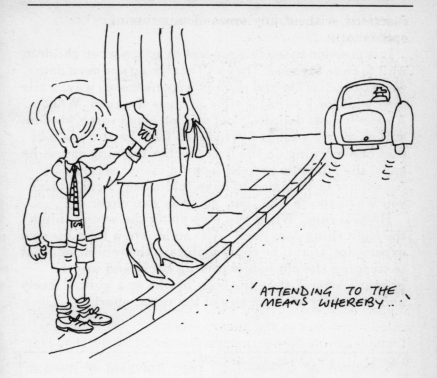

ATTENDING TO THE
MEANS WHEREBY...

Alexander called this kind of problem with our feelings 'faulty sensory appreciation'.

'Inhibition'

Recognizing this problem led Alexander to the third discovery. This was that before he did something, he had to stop so he could work out what he needed to do in order to carry it out well. This discovery of the need to stop he called 'inhibition'.

This turned out to be an unfortunate choice of words. Alexander made his discoveries before Freud's writing had become popularized and translated into English, but from then on 'inhibition' has been popularly thought of as something to do with the artificial supression of emotions and behaviour. Alexander, however, used the word in its physiological sense, meaning a healthy and natural self-control of unwanted and inappropriate reactions, without any sense of suppressing spontaneity.

It is possible to see this concept in action when children wait to cross the road. They will chat, sing and even dance, wave to each other and so on in a spontaneous way, while they wait for a suitable time to cross the road. What Alexander was definitely not talking about was a wooden, stiff or overly serious attitude. In fact the story is told that one morning on the first teacher training course he gave, the students arrived looking rather serious. Alexander is supposed to have told them, 'I can't teach you when you're like that; go away and cheer up!'

He also said, 'When you stop doing the wrong thing, the right thing does itself.' Alexander knew from his own experience, that if he could maintain the inhibition, that is stopping the old habits coming back, and use the primary control, then the body moved and worked freely and naturally without any of the usual effort.

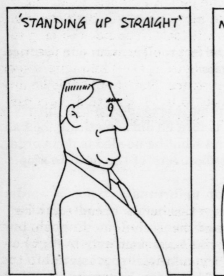
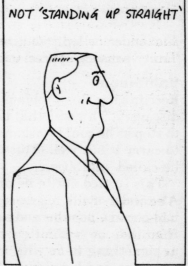

'WHEN YOU STOP DOING THE WRONG THING, THE RIGHT THING DOES ITSELF'

TOWARDS A SOLUTION

When Alexander found a way of integrating these
discoveries in practice, he had found the answer to his
problems. By recognizing the strength of his habits and
the inappropriateness of 'end gaining', he was forced to
look carefully at what he was doing and consider the
'means whereby' he was going to gain his end. In this
process he had to overcome his 'faulty sensory
appreciation' of how his body should be. This he did by
'inhibiting' his initial 'end gaining' way of working and
instead, by ensuring he kept his 'directions' for operating
the primary control, caused the body to work more
naturally.

Like the kerb drill learnt by children this process
requires repetition and time. Trying to force things to
happen or going too quickly simply excites fear reflexes
which block the possibility of free, natural body use.
Instead we have to give time for the conscious thoughts
of the directions to be laid down in the nervous system.
This in turn will affect the general muscle tone, and
through this, posture and movement will both change.

It is not surprising that it took Alexander so long to
make his discovery and perfect the Technique in practice.
Even with this written information, the Technique is very
difficult to carry out in practice. Nor should this be any
other way – no one expects to learn how to drive a car,
for example, or play a musical instrument from just
reading a book.

THE TEACHER'S ROLE

The work of the Alexander teacher is, of course, to be
able to explain the ideas of the Technique and help to
diagnose the student's problems and then to find out how
to deal with them. But beyond that, what is vital to the
student's learning of the Technique is the skilful use of
the teacher's hands to give the experience needed. This
way of using the hands is achieved by a long period of

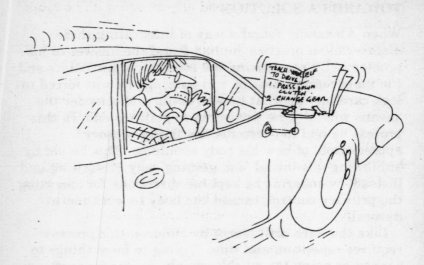

NOONE EXPECTS TO LEARN HOW TO DRIVE A CAR OR PLAY
A MUSICAL INSTRUMENT FROM JUST READING A BOOK

training in which the teacher becomes so fluent in the
Technique, that they are able to use and apply the steps
Alexander discovered reliably to themselves. The result
is that they have a quality of muscle tone in their body
that allows them to transmit the same possibilities to
the muscles of the student. As a result the student can
be helped, not only to observe themselves and understand
what is being attempted, but above all to *experience* what
changes can be achieved and the quality of body use
required to gain these.

ALEXANDER'S METHOD

Let us go back and look in more detail at the actual process
Alexander went through to make and integrate his last
three discoveries. After much experiment he found that
he had to fool his brain to prevent it telling the muscles
to get ready in its old habitual way. For example when

he got ready to recite, instead of 'just doing it', he found that he had to:

1. refuse to do it immediately (inhibit);
2. give the directions for the primary control in sequence;
3. keep giving the directions until he was confident that he could use them to do whatever he wanted to do (that is he was attending to the means whereby);
4. while still sending the directions, he stopped and reconsidered what he actually wanted to do. He then made a fresh decision to be equally open to either
   a. doing something completely different or,
   b. going on to do the action or,
   c. doing nothing at all.

In each case, when he made his new decision he continued repeating his directions, that is consciously wishing his neck to be free, his head to go forward and up and his torso to lengthen and widen. These directions provided the 'means whereby' his body would work with the maximum ease and effectiveness as they operated the primary control.

This may sound a difficult and complicated procedure but, with the expert help of a teacher this essential practical skill is made much easier. The teacher can, by means of his hands, enable the student to experience the primary control working, while at the same time learning how to give the corresponding directions. Because the teacher has a very acute sense of what is happening in the student's muscles from his hands, he is able to ensure that the student really does keep the primary control working well during the action. Should this be lost at any time, the teacher can stop the student and take him back to the point where he lost it, so the student can pinpoint his problems and learn how to overcome them.

This is a gentle, delicate process involving non-judgemental awareness on the part of both teacher and student, combined with great attention being paid to what is actually happening. This very accurate observation and clear diagnosis, together with positive and practical help in the solution of difficulties, is the hallmark of good teaching.

4.
THINKING ABOUT ALEXANDER TECHNIQUE

What exactly is the Alexander Technique? Why do I need it? How many lessons do I need? How long does each lesson last? How can I find an Alexander teacher? How do I know if they are properly trained? What do lessons cost? What should I wear? These are just a few of the many questions people ask when considering whether or not to consult an Alexander teacher and in this chapter I will attempt to answer them, and some of the others that crop up regularly so you can approach the Technique fully informed and confident.

What is the Technique?
Briefly, it is a practical method for finding out what habits of body use we have and how we can prevent those which we find to be harmful.

Why do I need it?
The instinctive body responses to danger are often triggered inappropriately by everyday events in our rushed, highly technological society. (Think, for example,

of the effect the noise of traffic has on you.) We become stressed and tense, and as a result pull our bodies out of shape. This pattern quickly becomes habitual, undermining not only performance but also health. The Alexander technique enables us to recognize such patterns *and* prevent them, allowing us to improve our overall functioning and general level of wellbeing.

What are the basic ideas?

Use: How we use our body affects how it can function. For example, trying to use a chisel as a screwdriver is a *misuse* of it, causing it damage and preventing it being used for its proper function of chiseling. Conversely using the chisel as it should be used and keeping it sharp will maintain its usefulness. Similarly our body will only work at its best if we learn how to use it correctly.

Inhibition: The process of stopping the misuse of the body is called inhibition. This involves a conscious refusal to act in the old way so that a new and better way of using the body can be found.

Sensory appreciation: To use the body well we have to ensure that it is accurately informed of what it is doing. Much of this information comes from proprioception. Due to bad habits of body use this sensory appreciation is faulty in most of us. With training it can be made more reliable.

Primary control: To improve our sensory appreciation we have to improve the way we use our body by learning how to activate the primary control. This is done by ensuring that all the parts of the body maintain a dynamic relationship with each other which maximizes the length and width of the torso and the ease of movement of the body as a whole. Although this is difficult to explain in words it can be quickly and effectively demonstrated by a teacher.

Directions: For Alexander the body was always being directed, consciously or subconsciously, well or badly, in a new way or habitually, to prevent something or cause it. In the Technique we are concerned, firstly to prevent misuse due to subconsious, habitual directions and then build up the primary control with consciously chosen directions, leading to a better use of the body.

End gaining: Going directly for what we want, acting immediately, without thinking of what we are doing in the process, is what Alexander meant by this term. He recognized it as a central problem in learning of all kinds, especially the Technique.

Attending to the means whereby: This is the key to stopping the over hasty reactions caused by end gaining, which are often the cause of misuse. Inhibition is needed to stop the end gaining reactions. New directions are then given to build up the means whereby the end can best be gained, step by step. In practice this usually means giving the directions that will build up the primary control.

How many lessons do I need?
Alexander prescribed a minimum course of 30 lessons. The number you need will depend on what you want to achieve and what problems you have. Mr G's symptoms improved in a matter of six lessons, although it took longer for him to learn the new use that prevented them from returning. For Diana K, on the other hand, the lessons were not undertaken to deal with any specific problems, and she took lessons intermittently over three years, using them to re-form her dance.

How long does each lesson last?
Alexander found that 30 minutes was the minimum time he needed to make useful changes. Today teachers use between 30 and 60 minutes. For most students this is the maximum time they can maintain the level of attention required and benefit from the changes which are occurring.

How can I find an Alexander teacher?

As advertising by teachers is restricted by their professional body you are unlikely to find lurid advertisements for them in newspapers and magazines. They may list themselves in the telephone directory under the Alexander Technique. The sure way of finding a teacher is to write to the secretary of The Society of Teachers of the Alexander Technique (STAT) whose address is at the back of the book (see p. 99) and they will send you a complete list of qualified teachers.

How do I know if a teacher is properly qualified?

A teacher should have a certificate issued by The Society of Teachers of the Alexander Technique (STAT), or by F M Alexander himself, or by one of the national societies of teachers now being set up in several countries. All these societies are affiliated to STAT and so a certificate from one of these societies should say this on it. If you are in any doubt contact the secretary of STAT.

What do lessons cost?

The price of a lesson will vary depending on the experience of the teacher, the length of the lesson, and their overheads. For example a practice in central London is much more expensive to maintain than one in the country. Fees range from about £15 to £40 in Britain, $20 to $60 in the USA and DM50 to DM120 in Germany, for example. There is no necessary connection between the quality of a lesson and the fee charged. If you can, I suggest you try two or three teachers before deciding who you want to work with and how much you want to pay.

What should I wear?

Ordinary, everyday clothes that are easy to move in are the best. Very tight jeans or very high heels are not recommended unless these are what you normally wear. I say this because the Alexander Technique is about how to live your *normal* life in a better way; it is not something that requires special exercises or clothing. You do not need to take your clothes off for a lesson.

Do I have to avoid eating and drinking before a lesson?

Only in as far as a heavy meal or too much alcohol can make you drowsy and less able to attend to the lesson.

Can I ask questions?

Yes!

What should I ask?

It is a good idea to clear up any basic queries before the first lesson, such as what are the teacher's experience, qualifications and fees. Also find out whether they think they can help you with your particular needs, and how often you should have lessons and how many. Ask what happens if you cannot do as many as they suggest. Find out if they are able to take you on now, or if they have a long waiting list. If they do, ask if they can recommend other teachers.

What should I tell the teacher?

It is a good idea to be as clear as you can about why you want lessons. What do you want to achieve? How much time will you have? If you have any particular medical problems be sure to mention them. Teachers will not wish to pry into your private life but, if you think anything of a personal nature is causing difficulties, it might be worth mentioning.

Additionally, if you read through the next sections and think you may have problems with the sort of things that happen in a lesson you should warn the teacher.

What will I be asked by the teacher?

Teachers usually like to have your home and work telephone numbers so that they can contact you if any changes of appointment are needed. If you are receiving

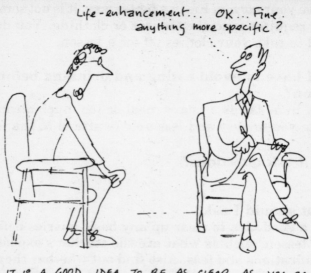

Life-enhancement... OK... Fine. anything more specific?

IT IS A GOOD IDEA TO BE AS CLEAR AS YOU CAN ABOUT WHY YOU WANT THE LESSONS

medical treatment they may ask you to check that your doctor approves of you taking lessons. If you have not discussed it already, the teacher will probably ask you why you want lessons and if you have any particular problems.

What happens in the first few lessons?

Exactly what happens depends of course on you, the teacher and your particular needs. What follows is only a very approximate guide based on my own experience. At the first lesson I generally sit down with a student and go through the various questions I have just indicated. When I feel we have got to know each other a little, I explain that I'd like to place my hands on the neck and shoulders as the student sits down, to feel what is going on. This gives me a rough idea of how tense the person is and gets us more used to each other. In particular it gives the student an experience of being touched in a non-invasive and non-judgemental way.

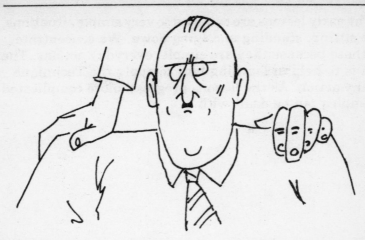

PUTTING MY HANDS ON THEIR NECK AND
SHOULDERS .... GIVES ME A ROUGH IDEA HOW
TENSE A PERSON IS ...

With one hand remaining on the neck I ask the student to stand up in the normal way. Having done this, we swap places and I copy the student's movement pattern, so he or she can see and feel what it is like from the outside. I then briefly explain what I saw in the pattern and how it is affecting their body. From this I go on to give a very brief outline of Alexander's discoveries and to demonstrate the effect inhibition and direction have on me. The difference is usually clear cut so that we can swap back. By using my hands, I can bring about the changes needed in the way the student uses his or her body so that they can feel the difference in themselves. Usually, students quickly feel that they are taller, lighter and move more easily.

As soon as it is possible, I ask students to start to think of the directions, so they can learn to use the primary control for themselves. In the early lessons this can only happen when my hands make the necessary change for them, but with time most students learn how to use it for themselves.

The early lessons are confined to very simple situations, like sitting, standing and lying down. We concentrate on these because they are simple, everyday actions. The aim is to help in learning how to apply the Technique to any action. As the lessons progress, more complicated examples can be dealt with.

5.
STAGES OF LEARNING

Each individual will vary in the rate they learn the Technique. Much depends on how much misuse their bodies have already received and how severe their problems are before the lessons start. Consequently, the following outline of stages is by no means definitive, although it does provide a general guide to the stages of progress experienced by students of the Technique.

FIRST STAGE

The first stage in learning the Technique is being able to experience the activating of the primary control through the teacher's use of her hands. In some students this is immediate – they can feel the changes in their musculature together with the lengthening and widening of their trunk. They feel lighter and freer when they move. Some will also report psychological experiences.

   The majority of students are a little slower in reaching the first stage. In my own case, although the early lessons were pleasant, I did not feel any specific or clear changes for about six months. However, most students do feel changes before then. In a few cases the student will not feel any changes at all. A senior colleague of mine tells of a man he was teaching, who had received 30 lessons and obviously did not feel anything. My colleague asked him why he was continuing to take lessons. 'Well', said the man, 'I've had to buy new jackets because I'm too broad for my old ones, I've also had to buy new shoes as my feet have grown and my children tell me that I'm a much nicer man to live with.'

This cautionary tale is important. It illustrates graphically the fact that the Technique is actually concerned with making objective improvements in the way we use our bodies, and that these objective changes may not be accompanied by any subjective changes. Alternatively, the changes experienced may not correspond to the objective changes. This is illustrated by a student who, when he was asked to free his neck, actually stiffened it. With another student, when I asked her to let her head go forward and up, she actually pulled it back.

These cases illustrate how our habits are deeply rooted in our ideas, our way of living and, in particular, in our way of responding to a demand being placed on us. Rather like animals when they sense something unusual, we automatically stiffen in response to a demand whereas, what is actually required in a non-survival situation, is that we remain quiet but alert for anything of interest. This allows us to respond in a free and effortless way. To help the students just mentioned, the trick was to ask them to think of stiffening and pulling the head back. This produced the respective freeing of the neck and releasing forward of the head! A further warning to be taken from these examples is the power of words. Each individual has his or her own personal set of associations for a particular word. This is especially true with habits.

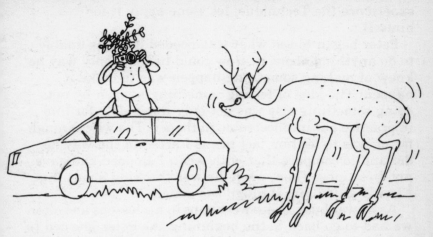

RATHER LIKE ANIMALS WHEN THEY SENSE SOMETHING UNUSUAL, WE STIFFEN..

SECOND STAGE

As the lessons proceed, and the objective changes are repeated with the help of the teacher, the student enters the second stage. In this stage the student begins to be able to give the directions for herself when she is still and the teacher's hands are on her. With some students this is a quick and simple matter. They are tuned in to their bodies and can, as Alexander phrased it 'ask nicely' for the greater freedom in their body use. However, for most of us, it is at this stage we meet the problem of habit. Take Peter F for example. He is a rock musician, whose work requires a lot of travelling, very hard and loud playing, and irregular hours. In his own words he is a 'go-getter'. His body is strong and in Alexander terms rather stiff and hard, a stance his body use reflected. His movements were very quick and rather angular, he was constantly ready to go. When we began working, I quickly realized that the problem we had to deal with was getting Peter to stop. Until he could be persuaded to stop, mentally as well as physically, he would be unable to experience the Technique, let alone apply it for himself.

Peter began to see what was needed but was unable to do anything about it. How could he? The only way he knew of making something happen was to make it happen! The idea of letting something happen by not doing something else was not only impossible for him in practice but inconceivable in theory. The way through for us was to let him feel me as I acted in the way he did and to compare that with when I stopped and gave my directions. Then, while he was thinking about this, I would guide him through the action.

As he was busy, there were gaps in his lessons and often we had to go back to the beginning. As Peter learned to stop and just leave his body alone, he began to experience the working of the primary control. Gradually, he was able to learn how to give his directions without trying to make something specific happen. Otherwise this usually resulted in either stiffening, or, if he tried to relax, a collapse of one part of the body, which makes it stiffen somewhere else. This led him to the third stage of being able to continue to give his directions when I guided him as he moved, for example, from sitting to standing.

THIRD STAGE

This third stage is similar to the stage Alexander reached when he found he could both give his directions and recite. The difference is that with the help of the teacher, the students are corrected almost automatically and as they go into action. This means that quite often, we do not have to explicitly teach the method Alexander used on himself to fool his habits at the critical moment of starting an action.

When students reached this stage with Alexander, he worked with them on two particular procedures. First, he concentrated on the process of bending forward, either when sitting or standing and putting the hands on the back of a chair. These he called the positions of

mechanical advantage or more familiarly 'monkey'.
Through working on this procedure systematically, a
student can learn how to do something with their hands,
be it writing, drawing, washing the dishes, adjusting the
controls of a car or playing a musical instrument, whilst
maintaining the primary control.

The second procedure was that of using the voice and
breathing to produce a particular sound, called 'the
whispered ah'. This leads to being more skilful in
anything that involves the voice or breathing, in giving
lectures, singing, talking on the phone or playing a wind
instrument, for example.

Between them, these two procedures provide useful
prototypes for studying the whole range of human actions,
from walking and running to dancing, cycling, jumping,
lifting, carrying, practising yoga, tai chi, or martial arts,
making expressive movements and to the study of body
language. Each of these deserves a book to itself but their
practice must be learnt from a teacher.

FOURTH STAGE

The fourth stage is one in which the student is able to
maintain the primary control without guidance in an
increasing number of activities and situations. At first,
it may only be possible in a reliable way in the teaching
room and only then for simple activities. As you gain in
experience this can extend outside to more and more
activities.

An example may help. Betty G is a secretary, an
amenable, efficient and helpful person. Her boss was used
to her being obliging and tended to ask her to work
overtime. Sometimes she resented this but she didn't
know how to say no. Her boss was rather overbearing
and she was rather timid. If she argued with her boss,
the boss always won.

One evening, when she was due to have an Alexander
lesson, her boss asked her to work overtime again. This
time, rather than saying yes or arguing, she gave her

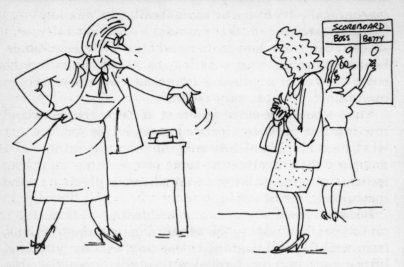

IF SHE ARGUED WITH HER BOSS, THE BOSS ALWAYS WON

directions, then, firmly but politely said, 'No, I have an important appointment.' The boss was so surprised by her straightforward polite refusal that she (the boss) had nothing to argue about and so had to agree. This saying no to old patterns by pausing and giving the new directions is equally effective in less emotional situations.

FAILURES

As with many areas of human endeavour, Alexander lessons sometimes do not work. This may be only a temporary hitch, we all have occasional difficulties in learning anything. Sometimes, however, it may be a more long term problem.

The most common problem is that of attitude. Occasionally, people who are sent to have lessons by well-meaning relatives or friends, are simply not interested. In other cases, the person is looking for a specific, quick and easy cure for their problem. They expect a teacher to sort them out with a maximum of speed and a minimum of interference with their normal life. In Alexander terms these people are 'end-gainers' who find this sometimes slow and painstaking work frustrating. They haven't got time for bothering about such things, they say.

Another problem of attitude, is sometimes found in people who are practising one of the various growth methods now popular. Before I go on, let me make it clear that I am in no way criticizing any of these methods but simply the fixed attitudes some people have towards a particular method. Some examples may illustrate these problems. Brenda A is a teacher who has suffered from neck and shoulder pains for some years. She took a form of posture training which taught her how to stand and sit correctly. Although the ideas themselves were sensible, they failed to deal with the habits underlying Brenda's neck and shoulder problems. When we came to work with each other, I found that as she got ready either to stand or sit, she would put one foot backwards first. This caused her whole body to stiffen and become noticeably shorter. We discussed the problem. I explained what I saw and felt in her body and demonstrated it. However, because it was such a part of her, Brenda did not feel it at first. The habit, especially because she had learned that it was the only way to move, was so powerful that no other possibility could even be considered. She could not allow herself the possibility of acting in a different way, not because she was resisting my work but because her feelings told her anything else was impossible. Gradually, as we continued our work, and I made it clear that I was not attacking the method she had learned but her response to it, she was able to take a fresh look at herself, and gradually learn how to let her body be free and light when she moved.

Robert J is a busy public relations officer for a large company. His work involves many meetings and planning conferences. He had developed an interest in psychology and various forms of psychotherapy, and through these he had made contact with some of the emotional factors in his life. He came to me for lessons as he was curious about the Alexander Technique. It was quickly apparent that Robert was over-relaxed, that is his body was very heavy and unresponsive. When I talked to him about this, he explained that he was feeling what was happening in his body and various emotions coming from our work together.

I explained that the focus of our work was attending in a more general way to what we wanted to do and what we were doing to ourselves in the process. As a part of that, feelings and emotions were important. However, if we concentrated purely on the feelings and emotions, we made it impossible to produce the improvements in the way we use our body and mind that, in turn, would have positive effects on our feelings and emotions. More generally, feelings and emotions tell us about what has happened or what we imagine might happen. They do not tell us what we can decide on or how we can achieve it. What we want is not to work against our feelings or emotions, but to have a clear perception of what is good for us.

Part of deciding is based on emotions: 'I want to do something'. The wanting provides the motive power. The how, the shaping of the wish, seeing how it fits in with a broader perspective, requires conscious thought. This is the aspect we are dealing with in the Technique. Robert agreed with this and I was able to demonstrate to him that his body could be lighter and freer with this new way of thought. However, this was not Robert's interest. He wanted to continue his exploration of feelings and emotions in his way, because this was what felt better and more important to him. This was his prerogative. The Technique is not concerned with conditioning or hypnosis or other methods of influencing people without their free will. It is concerned with the use of observation and choice and people must be free to exercise these facilities.

One reason students give for stopping lessons is money, or rather the lack of it. I would suggest, that if this is

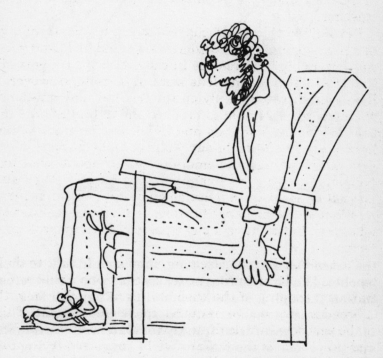

IT WAS QUICKLY APPARENT THAT ROBERT WAS
OVERRELAXED AND HIS BODY HEAVY AND
UNRESPONSIVE.

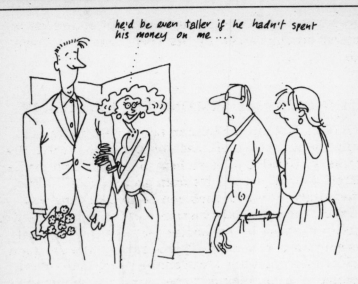

he'd be even taller if he hadn't spent his money on me....

THE REASON STUDENTS GIVE FOR STOPPING LESSONS IS LACK OF MONEY.

the reason for anyone stopping, they should talk to their teacher. I know of no Alexander teacher who would refuse tuition through a student's inability to pay full fees.

Sometimes a teacher fails to 'speak the student's language'. It is difficult frankly to relate well to everyone and this is one of the reasons why I suggested trying two or three different teachers before you decide with which one you want to study.

WHY IT TAKES A LONG TIME TO LEARN

As you can see from the examples given so far, there are real problems to overcome in learning the Technique. Psychological and physical restrictions are so intertwined as to be inseparable. This is why Alexander talked about the 'self' rather than mind or body. Such problems cannot be solved quickly, they are part of ourselves. Instead we have to allow growth and development to work. This allows us to integrate the psychological and physical changes brought about by the Technique at our own pace.

WHY INDIVIDUAL LESSONS ARE NECESSARY

Each of us is a unique human being with individual requirements. Above all, each of us has to receive the necessary stimulus to learn how to use our own primary control. We can learn a lot from groups, most of the material given in this book can be taught that way. However, the essential experience of the primary control actually working in our bodies requires the physical intervention of a teacher. This is rather like tuning a musical instrument or a car engine; each individual instrument or engine has to be physically adjusted for it to work well. The very complexity of our body-mind makes this a demanding and delicate task. This is one of the reasons for the long training of teachers and the need for the sensitivity in the use of their hands. The process of adjustment is intensely personal, it needs time and a supportive, unstressed situation. Further, much of what is exchanged between student and teacher is private. The confidence needed to allow the fundamental changes required by the Technique often needs the confidentiality of private lessons.

There is a place for group work in the Technique. With my students I like to have monthly group meetings where we can discuss the Technique, new information can be given, and some practical work done. However, this requires continuing individual work to ensure each person can take on board whatever practical changes are suitable for them.

WHY 'HOW TO DO IT' BOOKS DO NOT WORK

Books, like groups, can inform, enthuse, and influence. 'How to do it' books, however, do not show *you* how to do it. Your particular needs and difficulties cannot be dealt with and it is precisely with these areas that the Technique is concerned.

6.
SCIENCE AND THE ALEXANDER TECHNIQUE

EARLY SCIENTIFIC SUPPORT

Some years after he arrived in England, Alexander had dinner with Sir Charles Sherrington, the greatest physiologist of modern times. Sherrington made some of the most significant discoveries on the way nerves control muscles and how the muscles are vital in informing the nervous system of what it should and should not do next. At a personal level the meeting was not a success. However, Sherrington supported Alexander's work for the rest of his life. He did this because he knew from his laboratory studies, and those of his colleague, Rudolf Magnus, that the neck and the head play a crucial role in the control of posture, balance and movement.

As he said, 'Mr Alexander has done a service to the subject [the physiology of posture and movement] by insistingly treating each act as involving the whole integrated individual, the whole psycho-physical man.

To take a step is an affair, not of this or that limb solely, but of the total neuro-muscular activity of the moment – not least of the head and neck.'

With the publication of Magnus' work in the 1920s, detailing the roles of the head and neck, physiologists and doctors who recognized Alexander's work began to speculate about the mechanisms of the Technique – how the body produced the changes we observe. Meanwhile, the number of physicians and surgeons seeing the benefit of the Technique increased to the point where 19 of them wrote a letter to the *British Medical Journal*, urging that the Alexander Technique be included in medical training.

EXPERIMENTAL EVIDENCE

The evidence lacking in all this was that of direct scientific experiment, although this requires much time and money. At the end of the Second World War, however, experimental studies did begin in Britain and the USA.

Doctor Barlow

In Britain, Doctor Wilfred Barlow, while in the army medical service, had begun to study young army recruits. These first experiments by Barlow were simple: a tape measure was hung from the back of the head; the length of tape between the back of the head and the bottom of the neck was measured, first when the person was standing and then when they sat down. During the process of sitting there was a shortening of the distance between these points due to the head being pulled back. The minimum distance was measured twice for each of 56 cadets and the average taken. All showed some shortening. Out of the total number of cadets, 45 had a shortening of over 1 inch and only 3 were aware they had shortened. Even when the cadets were asked to focus on the shortening, only 12 could feel it. When asked to stop the shortening from happening, only 7 were able to do so. 39 still had shortening of over 1 inch even though they thought that they had not shortened. This clearly demonstrates Alexander's point about the inaccuracy of our feelings, and the fact that we cannot make something happen just by trying when our feelings are so inaccurate.

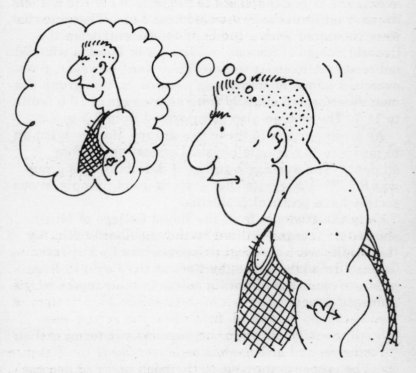

FEELINGS CAN BE INACCURATE — SOME
THOUGHT THEIR NECK HAD NOT SHORTENED
WHEN IT HAD . .

By asking subjects to stand in a standard position using a method developed by Professor J M Tanner, Barlow photographed a person from the front, side and back. He was able to analyse their posture from these photographs and reliably score the quality of their posture.

Barlow gave lessons to a group of 40 students from the Royal College of Music in London. They were photographed in the standard position before and after the course of lessons. Before the course the men had an average of 11 faults and at the end only 5. For the women the average faults were reduced from 9 to 4. These results were compared with a group of 44 students from the Central School of Speech and Drama in London who did not receive Alexander lessons. They were, however, given exercises aimed at improving posture. In this group the men deteriorated slightly from an average of 10.6 faults to 11.7. The women also deteriorated from 7.5 to 7.9.

As a comparison to these two groups, Barlow went on to measure 112 female physical education teacher students. The average number of defects in this group was 8.5. This suggests that even fit young people in our society have postural problems.

Only the students from the Royal College of Music showed an increase in height and shoulder width. All the results were assessed independently by Professor Tanner. In addition the teachers at the Royal College of Music made the following points in their report on the students' progress:

1. All the students improved physically in terms of their singing and acting abilities.
2. The students were easier to teach and had become more psychologically balanced.
3. The rate of improvement varied greatly between students.
4. The success of the students in an important singing competition was far greater than could have been expected.

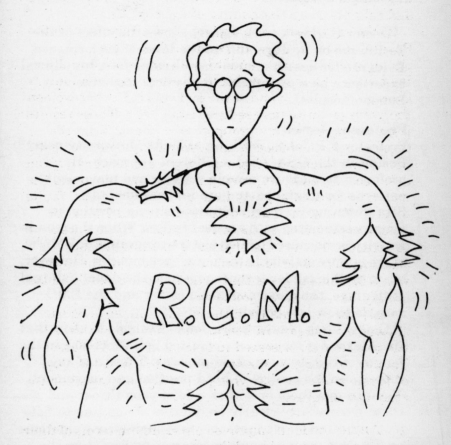

ONLY ROYAL COLLEGE OF MUSIC STUDENTS
SHOWED AN INCREASE IN HEIGHT AND
SHOULDER WIDTH...

5. In their opinion the Alexander Technique was the
    best method they had experienced for helping a
    singer's performance and should form the basis of a
    singer's training.

Doctor Barlow's work clearly shows the effect of the
Technique on posture and on the level of performance.
Evidence for health improvements came from his clinical
experience as a consultant in physical medicine at a
London hospital.

Professor Jones
Professor F P Jones, working at Tufts University near
Boston in the USA, used a different approach. He
preferred to measure muscle activity and movement
patterns for unguided and guided movements.
Straightening up from a slumped sitting position is
usually associated with a sense of effort. When the muscle
activity is measured (called electromyographs or EMG's),
there is more activity in the main neck muscles. However,
when an Alexander teacher prevents the usual habitual
stiffenings, the movement feels easier and the EMG
records show less activity.

Using X-ray photographs, Jones was able to show that
the Alexander movements resulted in an increase in the
length of the sternomastoid muscles. These are key
muscles in the control of head position and movement.
You can feel them on either side of your throat and see
them particularly clearly on dancers struggling to hold
a position and on actresses trying to show strong emotions
on TV soap operas. Another interesting find from the X-
ray photographs was that there was an increase in the
width of the discs between the neck vertebrae in
Alexander subjects. Also, the X-rays showed a forward
movement of the centre of gravity of the head. In other
words an Alexander subject was taller, her neck was freer
and the head had moved forward and up.

Jones used his techniques on the movement from sitting
to standing. His movement photographs show a quicker

and more direct movement. Unfortunately, he did not publish records of the muscle activity during the movement. Professor Finn Boyson-Møller of the University of Copenhagen and I therefore repeated the experiments using movement photographing equipment developed at the University of Copenhagen. In this experiment we also used a force platform. This is a piece of equipment which measures the size and direction of forces on it. Professor Jones had used one, but not in combination with the photographic and EMG measurements. Carrying out simultaneous recordings has the advantage of showing how these three measurements are related.

Our measurements showed that a guided movement required less force, used less muscle activity and was smoother and quicker than the habitual.

One problem with using photographic techniques is that slow movements are lost and taking measurements from the photograph leads to errors. For these reasons I went on to use a new electronic movement measurement system called Coda 3. The results of a pilot study allowed me to measure the speed and direction changes between someone moving in their habitual way, then trying to move faster and then using the Alexander Technique without guidance.

The results showed that using the Alexander Technique gave a more consistently upward movement with less wasted downward and backward movements of the body. As a result the movement took less time and force. In short it was more efficient.

Startle pattern

In other experiments Professor Jones studied the startle pattern. This is the typical reaction of someone when they are startled, for example, by a sudden unexpected noise. Jones found that the pattern always began in the neck and spread down the muscles of the body. It retracted the head, raised the shoulders, flattened the chest, straightened the arms and bent the legs. When one looks

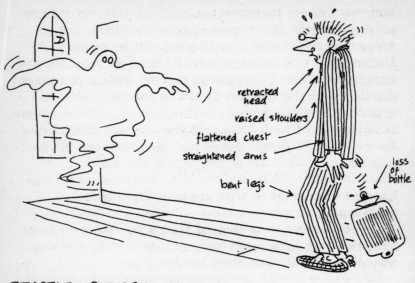

retracted head

raised shoulders

flattened chest

straightened arms

bent legs

loss of bottle

STARTLE PATTERN

at people in the streets, it would seem that the startle pattern is more and more the norm for people as they get older. The balance of the head is changed, the neck is shorter and pulled forwards. The head is pulled backwards by the sternomastoid and trapezius muscles, just as these muscles tensed in the habitual movements shown earlier.

Sway analysis
What happens to our balance if we prevent this stiffening? A good measure of this is what is called sway analysis. When we stand, we do not stand still, we sway a little. Usually, this is not noticeable, but if we are drunk or have damage to some parts of the brain, the sway becomes exaggerated. Using a force platform we can analyse the sway, how much, how fast. At the University of London Dr Roger Soames and I have investigated the effects of the Alexander on sway. We found that experienced Alexander students were significantly more stable than untrained subjects. There were also marked differences in walking.

Moving the centre of balance

As you can see from the various drawings the result of Alexander lessons is usually a more upright standing position and it is evident that the body is more aligned. This was checked in detail by Dr David Garlick at the University of New South Wales in Australia. He found that Alexander lessons move the centre of balance of the body backwards, confirming Barlow's and my findings.

QUALITY OF PERFORMANCE

Doctor Barlow's study with students singing showed that there was a correlation between the objective posture changes and the reports on the students' performance from their professors. Jones was able to show that not only did a singer and others listening to her feel that the voice and breathing were improved, but there are measurable objectives changes in the sound as recorded by spectral analysis.

BLOOD PRESSURE

Both Jones and Barlow report cases of reductions in blood pressure in hypertensive students. To look more closely at this in normal subjects, Michael Nielsen of Aarhus University in Denmark and I carried out experiments on musicians under stress before and after Alexander lessons. These showed a significant drop in blood pressure.

BREATHING

Doctor Barlow found the Technique useful in dealing with breathing problems. Doctor Garlick and his team have investigated breathing and found that it is deeper and slower in people who have had Alexander lessons.

In the USA Dr John Austin measured both lung capacity and the maximum rate at which people could breathe out, the latter being a very good measure of how well the lungs are working. Both measures showed a significant improvement after a course of Alexander lessons.

DIGESTIVE PROBLEMS

Doctor Barlow found that the Technique helped with various disorders of the digestive system. No experimental studies have yet been published, but Barlow's clinical findings, and those of other doctors, confirm cases reported by Alexander. Alexander hypothesized that the problems helped by the Technique were caused by the high pressures from narrowing and pulling down, producing a downward movement of various internal organs. By restoring the length and width of the torso, the Technique makes possible the return of these organs to their normal positions and functioning.

Much work remains to be done to investigate the effects of the Technique more thoroughly. To this end the Alexander Research Trust has been set up and appeals for donations to fund further research. This is important for several reasons. Firstly, by documenting the benefits of the Technique, its usefulness will be more widely appreciated. Secondly, uncovering how the Technique achieves what it does will help us to understand it better. As a result we may find more effective ways of teaching it and contribute to a deeper understanding of the human being.

Already the experiments I have done have enabled me to find improved ways of teaching the Technique. This is because the sensitivity of modern scientific instruments allow us to clarify and deepen our understanding of Alexander's discoveries. Using such instruments sensitively allows us first to repeat his work with even more precision and discipline, and then to make new developments. A possibility he looked forward to in his last book.

7.
HOW CAN I HELP MYSELF?

Part of learning the Technique is finding out how to apply it to our own lives and interests. In this chapter I have sketched out some ideas about ways of doing this and I hope you will find them a useful addition to the practical work you do with a teacher. Throughout this chapter I am assuming that you are taking or have taken Alexander lessons. (This is in no way meant to be a 'how to' book.)

LYING WITH THE HEAD ON BOOKS

Most teachers will, as a part of at least some of their lessons, teach lying with the head on books. Please note, that this is not how we suggest you go to sleep. We use this procedure to give the maximum possibility for bringing the body into good shape. All that is needed is a warm room, a table covered with a blanket or a piece of carpeted floor and some paperback books. The principle of the exercise is, that by supporting the body on flat firm

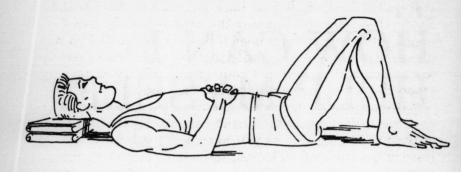

LYING WITH THE HEAD ON BOOKS

surfaces, the muscles not only relax but the shape of the body changes, allowing the spine to lengthen, the ribs to widen and the head to rock forwards on the top of the neck.

What height of books do I need?
The number of books needed depends on your height and the size of your spinal curves. The easiest way of getting a rough idea of how many books you need is to stand normally with your bottom and shoulders against a wall, then measure the distance between the back of your head and the wall. If you add 1 inch to this distance that is the approximate height of books you need. Your teacher can give you more precise information.

How to lie down
As you will have found out in your lessons just doing something always causes shortening. Instead you need to pause and give your directions. It is useful to experiment with different ways of lying down to avoid building up rigid habitual ways of trying to do it right. When you are lying down in the position shown in the illustration above stop for a moment and instead of trying to get comfortable, remember the problems of

blindly trusting your feelings. Rather just let your head
rest on the books and your back rest on the table or the
floor. Allow yourself to enjoy the experience. By this I
do not mean pretend it is good if it is not. If you feel pain,
please talk to your Alexander teacher and if necessary
see a doctor. If you are not comfortable after you have
stopped, then do move and repeat the stage.

Without losing your sense of enjoyment and your
awareness of the back and head being supported, think
of the neck being free as you have learned from your
lessons. As the neck releases, the head, relative to the
neck, is rocked forwards by the upthrust from the books.
Just give permission for this to happen. The result of the
neck releasing and the head going forwards is the
lengthening of the spine and widening of the torso. In
a lesson situation the teacher's hands bring this about.
When you are on your own, it is your own giving of the
directions that makes this possible. Of course, in a lesson
the teacher's hands are used to help you give the
directions but they are not a substitute for you giving
them. Other directions that are useful are for releasing
and lengthening the arms and legs (these will be taught
by your teacher when you are ready). The important thing
to remember here is not to concentrate on any particular
part of the body. The primary control has to be kept
operating while we extend our attention to include the
limbs. Don't forget the primary control and only think
of the limb you are working on.

SITTING

Sitting puts more stress on the spine than standing, so
it is not surprising that people who sit a lot, particularly
if they drive, are liable to back pain. How you sit can
have a big effect on your chances of avoiding pain. Sitting
slumped, particularly if you are leaning forwards,
increases the pressure on the discs of the spine. Having
lessons in the Technique will help reduce slumping
considerably. Working with your teacher on the

particular demands of your work and interest can help
with these areas of your life.

If you have to sit for long periods, you may find the
concept of the pelvic support useful. This idea was
developed by John Gorman, an engineer, who suffered
from back pain. His reasoning is interesting, even though
it is not generally accepted as yet. When we sit in a
balanced way on a hard flat surface our pelvis and lower
spine are roughly in the position shown in diagram A
opposite. If, however, we are tired, we slump. This is
the typical position people come to if they sit unsupported
for any length of time (see diagram B, opposite).

Unfortunately designers and ergonomists have
mistaken this habitual posture, due to misuse and
fatigue, for the natural. Accordingly, they have designed
seats to fit this pattern. Although there have been some
improvements, at least in car seat design, in recent years,
most people sit as shown in diagram B opposite, even
in well-designed seats. This is because of the strength
of their earlier habits and the lack of support for the
pelvis. Diagram C opposite shows a typical example.
Compare this with diagram D on the same page, where
a pelvic support is used. The difference in the curve of
the lumbar spine is obvious, particularly at the bottom.

As most slipped discs are in the lower two joints of the
lumbar spine, it is tempting to suggest that correcting
the lumbar curve will prevent such damage in the spine.
For more active sitting it is often better to do away with
the back rest. Using a firm chair which can tilt forwards
about 10 to 15 degrees, helps in stabilizing the pelvis.
Raising the seat height so that the angle between the
trunk and the thighs is about 120 degrees helps
further.

What needs to be stressed is that it is important not
to force yourself to sit up straight. A famous French horn
player found this to his cost. Knowing from experience
the importance of good posture for playing his instrument,
he had always prided himself on sitting up straight.
Unfortunately, this was actually sitting up stiff and the

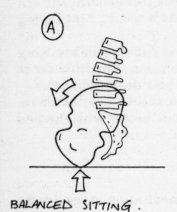

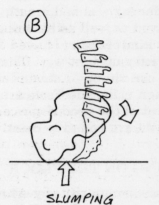

BALANCED SITTING.

SLUMPING

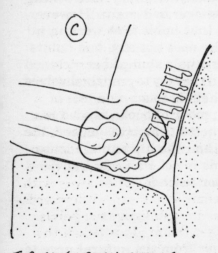

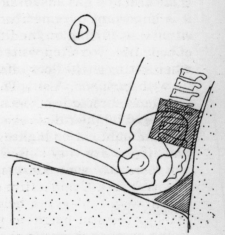

TYPICAL 'NORMAL' SITTING
IN A CHAIR OR CAR SEAT

SITTING WITH A PELVIC
SUPPORT.

result was two slipped discs. Forced to reconsider, he took Alexander lessons and found how to sit freely. Also, he saw that his back problem was a part of general pattern of stiffening and that another part of this general pattern of stiffening was bad breathing. As a result, his playing improved as well as his back.

The kind of chairs I have talked about are aids to sitting in an easy upright way. They are not a substitute for it – you can slump or strain in the best designed chairs. Through using the Technique you will be able to make the best of the good chairs and cope better with the bad ones you are bound to meet.

SITTING ON THE FLOOR

With the popularity of yoga and meditation many adults like to sit on the floor, as do many children. Such sitting is natural and has advantages over bad chairs. However, it is important to remember that habit is at work in all situations. Sitting on the floor does not stop bad habits of body use. Too often we see people slumped or strained when sitting on the floor, often they try to prop themselves up with cushions. A simple help is to sit on a pile of telephone directories. The number of books needed can be judged by the rule that when sitting cross-legged, the knees should not be higher than the hip joints. Please note, if you are very stiff, this is not true and I advise you to consult your Alexander teacher.

EXERCISE

Doing sport or exercises comes from the natural urge to move. Animals in the wild do not need them, neither do so-called primitive peoples. This is not surprising, as moving quickly and well is essential for survival in nature. As humans have become civilized, they use their bodies less and less. Thus there is an argument for doing exercises to give the body a chance to 'work out'. The problem is that not only have we underused our bodies,

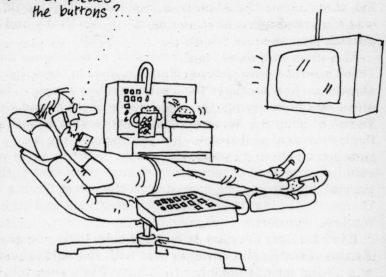

I don't suppose you also make a robot that presses the buttons? ....

AS HUMANS HAVE BECOME MORE CIVILISED THEY HAVE USED THEIR BODIES LESS.

but we have also learned to misuse them. If we don't deal with the misuse and eliminate it, we will exercise the misuse along with our body. It is like trying to drive a badly maintained car, something is going to go wrong. You have to stop and mend the defects as a first step.

For athletes who have used the Technique the result has been an improvement in their performance and a reduction in injuries. Take Paul Collins, an international level marathon runner, who represented his country at the 1952 Olympic Games. Knee injuries forced him to stop running for many years. Later, he came across the Alexander Technique and after having lessons, he noticed that his knees were better. He began running again and now at the age of 60 holds world records in running for veterans.

Howard Paine was an Olympic level hammer thrower. At the age of 40 he thought he was 'over the hill'. He, too, came across the Alexander Technique. The result was a marked increase in the length of his throw and a greater enjoyment of his sport.

At a more mundane level a number of colleagues and I took running lessons from Paul Collins. In these he showed us how to apply the Technique to running. The effect was electrifying: the usual sense of effort and slog vanished, running became a joyful expression of our bodies' natural abilities, rather than something we imposed on them by willpower. At an objective level we could see the kind of movement change from that of the normal runner you see everyday in the street forcing themselves along, to the style of Steve Cram and other top level runners.

Exercise does not have to be strenuous to do you good. Recent research shows we do best with the equivalent of walking for one hour a day. Elaine T is a research chemist whose boyfriend likes fell walking. He is tall and long-legged whereas Elaine is short and plump. When they first met, she naturally wanted to share his interest, but found she could not keep up with him. For quite different reasons she began taking Alexander lessons and coincidentally discovered that walking became easier and easier and that she could do a full day's walking and keep up with her boyfriend without undue fatigue.

Swimming is another area to which Alexander exponents have applied the Technique. Tony Buzan, who lectures internationally on how to use your brain better, is also an experienced long distance swimmer. When he learnt the Technique it changed the way he swam. Instead of fighting the water his strokes were smoother and more effective. In particular giving the directions allowed him to move his head much more easily for breathing and the breathing itself became easier and fuller.

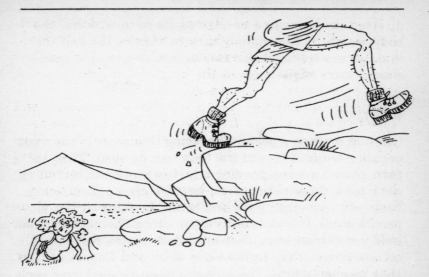

ELAINE IS SHORT AND HER BOYFRIEND IS TALL. THEY BOTH LIKE FELL-WALKING BUT SHE COULD NOT KEEP UP WITH HIM.

LIFTING AND CARRYING

We cannot avoid lifting and carrying, but we can avoid some of their harmful effects. In the course of lessons you will almost certainly be taught the position of mechanical advantage, or as we call it, monkey. Learning this position (or more accurately movement) gives you a chance to apply the Technique to any situation requiring power. It is the position humans naturally go into when they get ready to do something needing effort. Tennis players waiting to receive a serve, runners at the start of a race, golfers and batsmen in cricket are just some examples. It is seen most often in daily life when someone gets ready to lift an object.

The problem once again is habit. The solution once again is observation, inhibition and direction. This can be demonstrated by the difference between the habitual and the directed use of the body in lifting. In most people (habitual use) the spine is distorted, the body weight is too far forward and the muscles are overtensed. In

93

directed use the spine maintains its natural form, the body weight is far enough back to aid the lift and the muscles are released and free to stretch giving a springy elastic start to the movement.

WRITING

Often, it is when a person is writing that some of the most peculiar ways of treating a body can be seen. This, in turn, causes a corresponding clutch of problems, including neck pain, frozen shoulders, writer's cramp, headaches, back pain, stomach pain and so on. Looking at the way people write, it is not really surprising. The neck is often held very tense, shoulders are lifted, people lean heavily on one elbow, they tighten the wrist and fingers so that they become white. The legs are often twisted over each other and the feet lifted off the ground or tapping up and down almost as though the person was wanting to run away. All of these nervous reactions can be prevented and the result is not only the end of the pain, but much better handwriting and increased pleasure in the task.

The overall solution to these, and many other everyday problems, is not some slavishly mechanical use of the Technique. Teaching body mechanics or good posture will not solve the problems. I was told of the following by a leading expert on back pain when his team was asked to help a company to train its workers in lifting. They observed the workers and saw that they were trying to bend their backs and hold their legs straight when they lifted things. So, the team trained them in good body mechanics, that is, keeping the back straight and bending the knees to lift. The result was a reduction in the number of cases of back pain but an increase in the number of people having knee pain – a good example of not seeing the real causes because of not understanding the message of the Alexander Technique.

What is needed is a sensitive and personal re-education of the individual to help them see how they are reacting

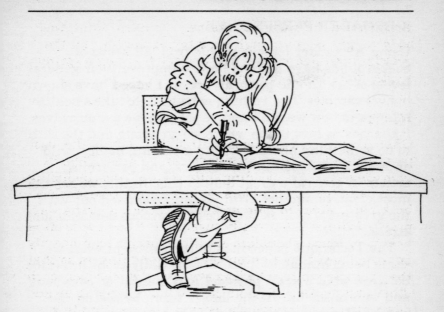

OFTEN IT IS IN WRITING THAT WE SEE SOME OF THE MOST PECULIAR WAYS OF TREATING OUR BODIES.

inappropriately to the demands placed on them and how they can find a practical way of responding in a better way.

REHABILITATION

One of the most important uses of the Technique is in rehabilitation after an illness, injury or operation. During this time the body is weak and needs the best possible chance to re-build and repair itself by improved balance, posture and movement. These, in addition to the usual rehabilitation methods, help reduce mechanical forces on damaged tissues and make recuperation a positive possibility for a new and better approach to normal life.

A BROADER PERSPECTIVE

Using Alexander lessons people from all kinds of backgrounds have learned how to improve their general levels of health and performance, as I hope I have shown in my examples. The Technique helps us to take a healthy interest in how we can improve the way we use ourselves. It teaches us how to see where we go wrong and the skill to do something about it. I find watching babies, wild animals, great sportsmen, dancers, and performing artists in general a great help in this. In this we see the most creative and powerful responses carried out with the greatest of skill in the face of enormous demands and stress.

The Technique penetrates to the centre of what we think being human is. It operates initially at the interface between what we call 'physical' and 'mental' or 'conscious' and 'subconscious'. In the longer term, by seeing the results of our conditioning and other environmental forces, we are faced with our ways of reacting to them and how we can prevent those reactions which are inappropriate. We are moving out of the fixed, subconscious and automatic towards a more conscious and flexible way of behaving. Although difficult to sustain at first, it becomes easier to the extent that it can be almost automatic but subject to choice. In short by developing conscious attention we become more able to choose and so deal with habits.

Too often we find ourselves stuck in a particular way of behaving based on fixed beliefs or fear. On the other hand 'changing' can be just as rigid a habit. It can be that the changes are just other ways of doing things badly and are an avoidance of the responsibility for making choices. In Alexander's own words, 'this work is about making choices and sticking to them against the habits of a lifetime.'

Because *we ourselves* are the instrument we must use, whatever we are doing, we need to know how to use ourselves well. As we develop this practical skill we are offered several possibilities. Firstly we gain in skill and health as has been shown. Additionally we can be more discriminating in our choice of activities as we have developed objective criteria for assessing whether or not they are actually beneficial. Thirdly we are able to develop the kind of dynamic constancy that is characteristic of well functioning natural systems. This gives the possibility of a more sensitive and constructive way of being which combines intelligence, flexibility, strength – and a good sense of humour! Through this we are given the opportunity to evaluate what we really want and how we want to behave. We then have the choice of working consciously with our own evolution, both inner and outer, with the tools Alexander has provided.

So far I have talked about the Technique in relation to ourselves but the implications of the Technique go far beyond this. Unbalanced and destructive behaviours caused by end gaining are to be seen in personal relationships, how we treat our children, medical care, education, politics, business and international affairs to name but a few. Perhaps it is clearest in the way we treat nature. In all these cases our old, blind, instinctive – or more accurately, habitual – ways of treating ourselves, other people and the planet are creating more and more difficult problems.

Alexander's discovery of what we do to ourselves and how to stop doing it, so we can perform whatever we do well, whilst preserving our health and sanity can, in my view, be extended to all these vital areas. By following Alexander's approach, we have the possibility of improving not just our individual state, but that of the world.

8.
TOWARDS
A NEW
MILLENNIUM

Near to the dawn of the twentieth century, Alexander had consolidated his discovery. This was before the great advances in scientific studies of the reflexes of posture and movement to be made by Sherrington and Magnus. One effect of this was to rob FM of the scientific background to improve the description of his technique and help in its further development.

Now, on the eve of the twenty-first century, we can move forward, bringing together the above with the recent great advances in science gives us new ways of building on Alexander's fundamental discoveries. But before getting too involved in this heady cocktail let's get our feet back on the ground.

ALEXANDER'S EXPERIENCE

You will remember that FM became an actor but developed voice problems which forced him to stop performing. Determined to find out the reason for his voice loss, he observed himself in a mirror when reciting and when talking normally to see if he could notice any behavioural reasons for his problems. After a long period of observation he realized that when he recited:

1. He was breathing in with an audible gasp.
2. He was adversely affecting the balance of the head on the neck.
3. He was exaggerating the curves of his spine, and there was undue muscle tension throughout the body.
4. This overtenseness was particularly noticeable in the legs and feet.

He found that 1. could be prevented by preventing 2. and 3. but that these in turn could only be prevented by inhibiting 4. first. This last point is of vital importance because he saw that the problems with his voice, breathing, head and neck were not to be solved in that area but by dealing with a 'something else' that was causing them. That 'something else' was the fact that he could not let his feet rest on the ground under the stress of reciting. In describing his discovery, Alexander said that he noticed that his feet were unduly arched with little real contact except for the outsides of the feet and toes, to the extent that his balance was adversely affected. [1]

He also found that the answer was not to 'just relax'; that made matters worse when he came back to trying to make improvements in his speaking practice. So, how did he solve the problems?

Alexander's answer
To one student struggling with such difficulties and trying to work out what he should do, Alexander aphoristically said, 'Be a good chap, just stop doing the wrong things first'. However, this leads to the questions: what are the wrong things I am doing? And even when I know what they are, *how* do I stop doing them?

Alexander's answer was – observe your behaviour, for example in a mirror, and find out for yourself. For more

on what he found take another look at pages 47 to 54.
Naturally, a competent teacher can be of great help, but
even then, without some more information it can seem
more difficult than perhaps it needs to be. Fortunately
we now have much more relevant scientific information
than was available to FM, so let's look at some of it now.

A NEW STARTING POINT: USING SCIENTIFIC DISCOVERIES TO BUILD ON ALEXANDER'S EXPERIENCE

Reflexes which support the body
We now know from scientific studies that the body is
supported by means of a series of reflexes, one of which
is the supporting reactions of the legs (and arms). This
reflex is triggered by contact with the skin of the foot (or
hand) and weight on the foot (or hand).

The different effects of the two was shown by
experiments where subjects' feet were put in icy water,
temporarily shutting down the nerves which serve the
skin. They were less steady than when their feet were at
a normal temperature even though the pressure on their
feet was the same.

Practice: We will not repeat what may seem to be an
unkind experiment! Instead from time to time notice
what you 'do' with your feet, for example when reading
this book or when sitting at a table. Many people tend to
contract their leg muscles and pull their feet up, either
completely or just leave their toes on the ground. You
can see this in the drawing on page 95. Inhibiting the
tendency to overtense the legs and feet allows the feet to
rest more easily on the floor and for the supporting
reactions to be triggered more effectively. More on how
to do this in other situations will be dealt with later.

The effect of being more conscious
Being conscious of this reality allows us to be more in
the 'here and now', which means that we are more

awake, and this enables the supporting reflexes to be more effective (and so give the body better support). It is interesting to note that these reflexes are turned off in normal sleep, becoming less effective when we become tired or fatigued. This is one reason why we slump when we are tired.

Practice: Observe the behaviour of sports men and women at moments of triumph and defeat. When things go well it is easy to be completely in the 'here and now'. It shows in the happiness on their faces, but look too at their posture. In triumph people are 'up'– body, arms and their legs can't help but support them, so much so that they often spontaneously jump for joy! Being truly in the 'here and now', as we are at the 'good' moments in life, is the most awake we can be, we will return to this several times.

Muscles which support the body
The effects of the supporting reactions in the legs and arms continue through the deep muscles of the hips, shoulders, trunk and neck. Thus we see how events in the legs and feet should have such an effect on the whole body.

   These deep muscles have special fibres which do not fatigue, unlike the fibres of the movement muscles which are usually nearer the surface of the body. So when the reflexes work well there is less of a sense of effort or heaviness in the body and the surface muscles show less activity. This allows the neck muscles, such as the trapezius and sternomastoid, to become less tense and so allows the balance of the head to return to normal as Alexander noticed.

Muscles which move the body
If we have interfered with the supporting reflexes, something has to hold us up and, like Pinocchio 'There are no strings on me', that something is going to be our own muscles. However, now these will be the

movement muscles (strictly we should say motor units)
which are good at producing movements but which
fatigue when required to keep on contracting for a long
period.

It would appear that it was this inappropriate triggering
of the movement muscle fibres which Alexander was
experiencing when he reported undue muscle tension
throughout the body. For it is these outer layers of
muscle that we can feel most easily and whose level of
tension we are most aware of. From my teaching
experience, this tension is one of the commonest causes
of chronic pain in the body.

Naturally there are other factors, such as anxiety,
emotional crises and overwork that can cause such muscle
tension and which may require other forms of intervention.
However, even in these circumstances, working in parallel
on the interferences with the support reflexes is, in my
experience, helpful in solving what may appear to be
different kinds of problems.

How the body can be pulled out of balance

The 'movement muscles' main function is to bend joints.
When such muscles are overactive we would expect to
see chronic examples of such bending.

Practice: To take Alexander's experience as an example,
if you contract your calf muscles you will see that the
heel rises and the toes flex, the combined effect being to
lift most of the sole of the foot off the ground. If you try
this with both legs when you are standing, you can
experience the interference with your balance.

If you now look in a mirror at the other parts of your
body, you can see the effects that over contracting the
lower legs and feet have on other parts of the body. If
you look carefully you may see that the shape of the body
has changed. Of course our example is a gross exaggera-
tion (I hope!) of normal responses to stress, but it gives
an idea of some of the problems we are dealing with.

For example, in compensating for being out of balance

many people contract the large and long movement
muscles of the back, causing it to stiffen and arch.
Also, this is what people usually do when they 'stand
(or sit) up straight'. Not only does the back stiffen and
arch, so does the neck. Look at the pictures, taken from
photos of the author. [2] In the first he does what most
people do when they 'stand up straight'. In this
'military' position you can see the arching of the back
and neck. Also notice that this makes him even shorter
than when he slumps in the second picture.

If you do this you will find that it is tiring. From the
foregoing it is not surprising – we are using the 'wrong'
kind of muscle fibres. It is noticeable that when people
do try to 'stand up straight' it doesn't last long and then
they slump – often even more than they usually do. As
Alexander himself once put it: 'I am putting into gear
the muscles which hold you up, and you are putting
them out of gear and then making a tremendous effort
to hold yourself up, with the result that when you cease
that effort you slump down worse than ever'. [3]

In this position the body is stiff and out of balance. This
is made use of in eastern martial arts, where it is well
known that such postures cause people to be easily
thrown or otherwise knocked to the ground. They further
recognize that such postures are to do with the whole
person being out of balance with their life and are not
'just physical'.

Why simple-minded relaxation is ineffective
It is tempting to think that a simple solution to this
problem would be to 'just relax'. Let's think for a
moment what this means. First we would feel where
we were tense and then relax those areas. But we have
already seen that the reason we are 'tense' is because,
in some way, we have interfered with the reflex
support system, *which we cannot feel directly.*
Remember this is a largely automatic system, but
which, according to Sherrington, is the most easily
interrupted of reflexes. [4]

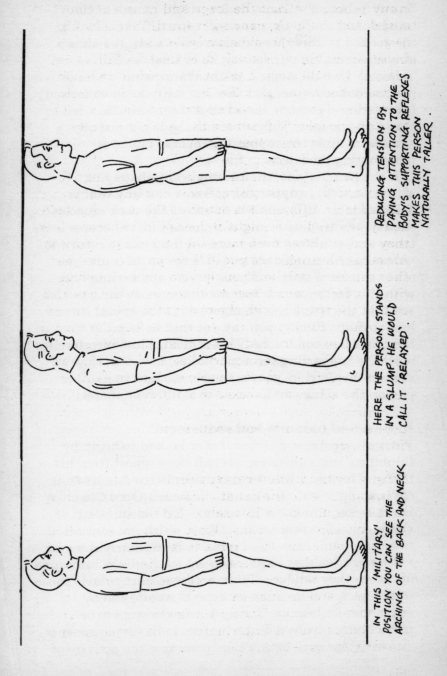

IN THIS 'MILITARY' POSITION YOU CAN SEE THE ARCHING OF THE BACK AND NECK.

HERE THE PERSON STANDS IN A SLUMP. HE WOULD CALL IT 'RELAXED'.

REDUCING TENSION BY PAYING ATTENTION TO THE BODY'S SUPPORTING REFLEXES MAKES THIS PERSON NATURALLY TALLER.

So our 'relaxing' will not deal with the causes of the
tension and so the tensions will return. Take a look at
the second picture; here the person stands in a slump,
almost normal in our society, he is what we call
'relaxed'. I would suggest it illustrates what we have
just been discussing, and that in reality he is 'collapsed'.
Interestingly enough, he is taller than when he tried to
stand up straight. This is because he is not actively
working against the supporting reflexes and so is
interrupting them less.

In the last picture, the person is simply paying
attention to the supporting reflexes in a way that is
detailed later. It is this which allows the neck muscles,
such as the trapezius and sternomastoid, to become less
tense and so allows the balance of the head to return to
normal as Alexander noticed. There can, of course, be
other causes of neck stiffness but we are dealing here
with this factor, which does seem common. You can also
see that the trunk has changed, with the spinal curves
less obvious. Finally you can see that he is taller than in
the other two conditions. This indicates less interference
with the supporting reflexes. Notice, however, that we
are not involved in 'good' posture, see how in another
person the spine can have quite a different shape.

Reflexes of balance and movement

We have seen how FM found that he had to begin by
inhibiting the interferences with the support from his
feet and legs and how we have scientific evidence that
this should lead to the results he found. Once the head
is not being pulled out of balance and the spine out of
shape, interferences with reflexes which are connected
to balance and movement seem to be similarly reduced.

Here are some examples of research findings into some
of these other reflexes. These reflexes, particularly those
in the neck and back, seem to be most affected by
Alexander Technique. The neck reflexes seem to be
particularly involved in the preparations for movements.
Twisting the neck to one side, increases the activity of

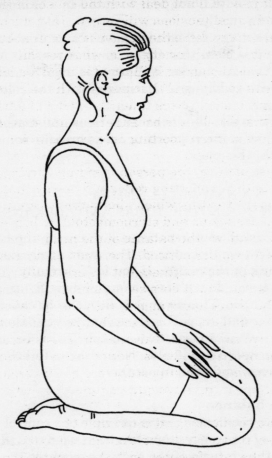

IN ANOTHER PERSON
THE SPINE CAN HAVE A
QUITE DIFFERENT SHAPE

the extensor leg muscles on that side – presumably to
prepare for the body to pivot on that leg as it turns in
the direction the head is looking. Bending the neck
backwards seems to cause both legs to tend to bend –
just what is needed if we squat down and still want to
look ahead of us. In the back it was found that the
sensitivity of the large surface lower back muscles is

107

important in both being able to stand in a balanced way and walk naturally.

There are many reflexes we have not covered but I hope that it is clear that there are good reasons for thinking that Alexander Technique is involved, at least in part, with reducing interferences with their good functioning.

In case this all sounds rather serious and mechanical, let's see how modern scientific ideas breathe some new life into things.

TOWARDS A NEW MILLENNIUM: MODERN SCIENTIFIC IDEAS AND ALEXANDER

Practice: Using your experiences of tensing the lower legs and feet we looked at earlier, start again standing and looking in the mirror. If you look carefully, you may notice that you do not stand completely still – in fact we all sway a little. This sway is believed to be caused by the balance and support reflexes actively rebalancing the body several times every second. This is because the body is unstable and is always tending to fall, first in one direction and then in another.

How we balance

This active rebalancing is an example of a control system. The idea of control systems has been used to understand many of the systems of the body, for example the control of the temperature of the body and the control of muscle contraction. In all of these, the system is never static; there is a constant slight variation in what is being controlled. We know about this sort of process from everyday life as the thermostat of a central heating system does not keep the temperature exactly constant. By careful design such systems keep the fluctuations so small that we don't notice them. This is the situation with our balance.

In the body, different control systems work together so the control of balance is connected to the control of muscle contraction. An example of this connection was found in the case of a surgeon who had problems with his hands shaking when performing operations. He realized that this was connected with the stiff postures he was putting himself in and took lessons from Alexander. As his control of posture improved his shaking was reduced.

This shaking is called tremor and is the result of a control system not keeping things exactly constant. When such a system is damaged or overloaded, the size of the fluctuation increases. This is what happens when the temperature of a central heating system does not stay constant. Tremor in surgeons' hands limits the fineness of the movements they can carry out and so the delicacy of the operation. For this reason research is now underway to produce mechanical arms whose artificial computer control system is designed to have a much smaller tremor and so allows surgeons to carry out operations that require a greater fineness of control than is possible with the unaided human hand.

Musicians (and others requiring fine hand skills) also have problems with tremor and one of the reasons that the Alexander Technique is so widely valued by musicians is the reduction in tremor it offers. As in music, where the beauty of a piece seems best expressed by a great artist, I find it more appealing to be operated on by a fully awake, well-balanced human than by a 'perfect' computer-controlled system. One reason is the ability of humans for 'lateral thinking', for creativity. More mundanely, in the operation situation, the human can notice something quite unexpected which throws new light on the problem being treated, and so on what they will actually do. We will look more at these abilities soon.

We can see the effect of interfering with our postural control system by observing the effects of drinking alcohol. From such observations it is well known that people sway more and have an unsteady gait. Experiments on sway using very sensitive equipment have shown that drinking even a very small quantity of alcohol increases sway. This increase is not noticeable to the person involved or to a casual observer, but shows up clearly on the equipment. This research is under-lined by a study on airline pilots. In this study, pilots who took alcohol were found to be able to react well to routine tasks but even small amounts of alcohol interfered with their ability to respond correctly to unexpected situations. This also supports the research of many scientists, and Alexander's experience, that the postural system has widespread links to many seemingly separate physical and psychological aspects of behaviour.

Practice: But back to you and the mirror, and sway of a healthier kind! Watch carefully as you decide to stand on one leg. You will notice that your body sways; try going onto the other leg, and your body will sway in the other direction.

What you may not be able to notice is that the sway begins *before* you lift one of your feet up. See if you see it when observing a friend trying the same exercise. If you look carefully you may see it. This only became clear when scientists began to use instruments which could look really accurately at the forces and movements involved. It was by using such instruments myself that I was able to look again at (re-search) what Alexander had discovered by looking in the mirror, but now with the improvements in sensitivity and comprehensiveness of coverage that modern technology makes possible. As a result of this experience and the enormous amount of relevant scientific information now available, I was able to find new approaches to the technique Alexander discovered.

When being unpredictable is good

Another factor in control systems which has only been discovered recently is that of its unpredictability. Let us return for a moment to the music played by a great artist as opposed to that on a computer. There is

something about the live performance which is more
appealing. This something, which is central to our
humanness is, in part, its unpredictability.

When a control system is interfered with, not only does
it fluctuate more but the fluctuations become more
regular. This is vividly illustrated in British guardsmen
who have to stand for long periods in a military position
while waiting for the Queen's inspection. This posture,
with its overcontraction of the muscles can interfere
with the supply of blood to the brain. This shuts down
the brain and with it the control of the balance and
support reflexes. This shows up in a gradual increase in
the sway of the guardsman, ending in him falling over.

It was not until the development of chaos theory that
we understood this. It turns out that a well-functioning
natural control system is marked by a *degree* of
unpredictability. It is just this *degree* of unpredictability
which we see in the weather, brain activity and heart
beat and – dare I suggest? – the behaviour of healthy,
gifted humans as shown earlier. Even we 'normal people' can enjoy new possibilities, make new discoveries,
even if these are as simple as deciding, on the spur of
the moment, to go home from work by a different route,
just for fun.

So we have this strange and fascinating combination
of regularity and persistence with openness to the new
and unexpected. This set of possibilities in our behaviour
is probably connected to the great development of the
brain, allowing us to imagine many possibilities and to
choose the most appropriate. By this we are not locked
in to what our genes and instincts dictate. How this
might work has been revealed in a series of elegant
experiments by Benjamin Libet and other brain
researchers. These were concerned with the way in
which the brain prepares for a movement. By using
sensitive measurement electrodes, brain activity before,
during and after a movement can be measured. The first
sign of electrical activity in the brain as a person
prepares for a movement is called the 'readiness potential'.

How we get ready to move

Preplanned movements: In 1964, scientists discovered this voltage (or readiness potential) in the outer parts of the brain (called the cortex) about one second before a movement we choose to make and can plan in advance, like deciding to pick up a cup in a few moments. This was underlined by other scientists in 1978 who found that, when a person only did a movement *in their imagination*, there was an increase in blood flow to the same brain areas as found by the earlier researchers.

Spontaneous movements: Libet found that a readiness potential (RP) is also set up in the cortex some half a second before a spontaneous movement begins.

. . . and inhibition: It appears that this RP begins about three tenths of a second before the subject is conscious of wanting to move. However, in the last two tenths of a second before muscle activity begins, the movement can be stopped. So even with a spontaneous 'decision', there is time for the person to choose whether to do it or not. In his experiments Libet showed that not only could his subjects change their minds, they could actually stop the muscle activity which would cause the movement from taking place.

Notice, however, that the preparation began in the brain *before* the person is conscious of having chosen to move. This helps us understand what Alexander was dealing with as he developed his technique for sensing and inhibiting postural and other habits. From Libet's work it appears there is a two tenths of a second period in which we can inhibit these after the spontaneous desire to move. Speaking of this process, Alexander said: 'You come to learn to inhibit and direct your activity. You learn first to inhibit the habitual reaction to certain classes of stimuli and second to direct yourself consciously in such a way as to affect certain muscular pulls.'

Practice: As you have experienced for yourself, before we lift a leg, there is a process of postural changes; in plain English we shift our weight.

Returning to the mirror, see what else you notice apart from the sway. Often people see that they bend and twist the trunk, others who are less steady will raise their arms and bend their head sideways. If you do not notice these changes try starting with the feet further apart. All these changes, and others are presumably to prepare the body for the new condition.

Improving movements

I was fascinated to see just how many unnoticed changes are made in the body before a movement when I used the very sensitive measuring equipment in my experiments.

In Alexander lessons, movements are often almost immediately improved when the subject is guided by the teacher. This has been measured photographically and by a force plate. Here the teacher helps to prevent the old habits from recurring and helps students to select new, more appropriate ones. As students learn this process, they also learn to bring about this improved pattern at will by improving their postural preparations (I confirmed this in my own experiments).[5] The idea of premovement postural adjustments may also go some way to explain the startle pattern referred to on pages 81 and 82.

Returning to the example of moving a leg, one function of muscles is to produce the movement and this muscle action is triggered by a command from the brain. Before this, however, the body prepares for the intended movement by moving the centre of gravity over the other leg. This is to maintain the equilibrium of the body. In addition, parts of the body will adjust their position relative to each other i.e. posture changes. Thus we see an interplay between movement, balance and posture.

Practice: Let's go on to something which is closer to everyday life, walking. Again stand in front of the mirror and start walking towards it. Did you walk straight towards it? I doubt it. If you observe carefully, you will see that the first movement you made was a sideways sway, just as you did when you went to stand on one foot. The scientific research into what seems such a simple act has found some quite unexpected things.

One such finding that is contrary to our intuition is that when we start to walk from a standing position the first movement of the body is backwards! This is because our postural support and balance system comes into play before the intended movement itself begins. We believe that this is connected with the readiness potentials in the brain and is largely unconscious and unnoticed (and often unnoticeable without using special instruments).

This kind of information shows us some of the reasons for support FM received from eminent scientists and doctors. In all our actions what we are doing *before* we do what we think we are doing, will have a great effect on the action and on the body in general. We can imagine how it is possible that if we build up chronic habits, these become built into the nervous system and so into the muscles; both those parts concerned with movement and those concerned with posture. These in turn lead to increases in the stresses on bones, joints, connective tissue, the systems of respiration, circulation and digestion, not to mention our 'mental state'; in short our whole self. Thus we gain a fresh understanding of Sherrington's endorsement of Alexander in which he said: 'Mr Alexander has done a service to the subject (the physiology of posture and movement) by insistently treating each act as involving the whole integrated individual, the whole psycho-physical man. To take a step is an affair, not of this or that limb solely, but of the total neuro-muscular activity of the moment - not least of the head and neck.'

Practice: Coming back to the mirror, you will also see that when you stand on one foot your sway increases, so much so that some people cannot stand on one foot for more than a few seconds. Part of the reason for this is simply to do with mechanics: the wider the base of support the more stable something is. But we nearly all stand on one foot as a part of daily life – as we saw earlier it is when we walk. So being able to balance, even with something as 'simple' as walking, is important.

More practice – improving balance: Let's begin with an easier situation – either standing on both feet or sitting. Now let's remember some of the things we saw earlier. The legs can best support the body when the feet are in good contact with a firm supporting surface. For example, try taking your shoes off so you can feel the floor more precisely. If you take a little time over this (sitting may be the most comfortable position) you can use your conscious attention to see how much information you can get from your feet; for example, the force from the floor supporting your feet. Can you distinguish between the contacts of the different toes, the ball of the foot and the heel? See what happens to these sensations if a friend gently touches those parts of your feet. Have them leave their hands gently but firmly on top of the foot, in front of the ankle joint to over the toes. Give yourself plenty of time to use this help to feel your feet on the ground more clearly.

With suitable help you should find that touch aids your perception, there are good reasons for this from scientific research.

Touch
Effects: Most Alexander teachers use touch to teach and guide movements. What does touch do? Touch, especially if it is unexpected, wakes us up. It is seen to change the blood flow in the cortex to that characteristic of greater alertness. Professor Jones found normal alert brain activity in Alexander subjects, further confirming that

the practice of the Technique is not like that of 'relaxation', on the contrary it is one of increased alertness.

Even light touch on the sole of the foot elicits the supporting reaction of the leg. Nerve cells specialised for sensing touch contribute to proprioception and give important background help for conscious movements. Such receptors on the soles of the feet were found to have a marked effect on balance, so we can see why working on letting the feet have more contact with the floor is important.

The role of touch in proprioception helps to explain why it is possible to feel more accurately what the body is doing during an Alexander lesson. This allows more efficient, easy and graceful movement. This news is good but when we see what conscious experience can add, the picture is even more positive.

Conscious experience of touch: Libet observed that when a subject's skin is stimulated electrically it takes about half a second for the brain to experience it consciously. However, the subject reports feeling the stimulus at the same time as it was administered. Libet hypothesised that the referral of the experience backwards in time was automatic. This is an important finding, for it had long been a puzzle as to how we seem to experience things in real time – that is when they actually happen.

In his most recent work, Libet has reported that the half-second delay occurs in the thalamus. This is a part of the brain below the cortex which is a vital relay station between the cortex and other parts of the nervous system. He also reported that some individuals were able to perceive the stimulation he was giving them (direct to the thalamus in this case) well before the half a second had elapsed. In some cases the recognition was almost instantaneous. It is as though the cortex is able to recognize a pattern well before it is fully formed. This is what presumably happens when we recognize someone at a glance, although of course we have all experienced being mistaken and having to look consciously to see if the person really is who we thought.

Pay attention!
Attention is probably a vital factor in such perception. A large number of investigations have been carried out into the effects of body feelings on the brain and comparing these with what the person experiences. The degree of attention the subject was able to bring to bear on a stimulus (in ordinary English, how conscious of it they were able to be) had a marked effect on the brain's responses and on the subject's ability to perceive the stimulus accurately. So we can see that it is reasonable to have the experience that being more conscious of our body allows us to perceive more things about it and that these feelings can become more accurate.

The problem is we know that it takes time for nerve impulses to travel from the sensors of the body (in this case nerves in the skin) to the brain. Also we knew that there were time delays in the brain before we could become conscious of the event. Thus, according to old-fashioned physiology, we could never experience the here and now. This meant that we could never make a conscious change to our behaviour in the here and now – we would always be too late. Some have even dismissed the idea of the existence of consciousness at all! Luckily the rest of us did not know this and carried on making conscious choices, as we have done for generations. A possible explanation of how we do the impossible on a daily basis comes, surprisingly enough from the hardest of hard science – quantum physics.

Beyond common sense
How is it possible for something to be experienced instantaneously? Under classical physics this is not possible, indeed according to one of its most powerful modern developments, Relativity Theory, the limit of the speed of transmission is that of light. Naturally, signals travel through nerves much more slowly than

this. Quantum theory, however, describes phenomena which have defeated classical physical approaches.

Quantum physics is concerned with the area of the very small – that is at the level of individual atoms and the particles which constitute them. When we reach these dimensions our common sense views of the world break down. So much so that one of the pioneers of quantum physics, Niels Bohr, had to explain to a colleague: 'Your ideas are crazy but not crazy enough for quantum physics.'

In our brains, individual nerve cells and sense organs, the areas in the cells where messages are sent from one cell to another, appear to be small enough to obey quantum rules. Let's see what some of these rules are. Quantum fields, unlike those we know – like gravity and magnetism – carry neither matter nor energy. They can also operate across any known distance instantaneously. These violations of common sense are so monstrous that Einstein and others devised an experiment to disprove such possibilities. Many years later technologies were developed which could make the test but the quantum predictions were not disproved.

Apart from any esoteric speculations, this allows the possibility of stimuli being consciously experienced instantaneously. It also suggests that the body is not a normal machine, whose actions are determined only by the normal, everyday laws of cause and effect. Instead there are only probabilities of things happening out of a multitude of possibilities. So vast is the number of possible interconnections and so complicated the connections themselves, that it is probably literally true to say that we have not even dreamt of most of them. Bohr's comment seems almost conservative after all that. However, the fact remains that the most powerful and (so far) successful form of science tells us that something can come from nothing, that in one sense the mind can be anywhere and yet exchange information with anything else, no matter where it is – instantaneously. No wonder humans can be so creative.

Once again let's get back to normal things, of the body and our experiences. The connection between consciousness and touch is enshrined in our language – 'Good to be in touch with you' we say to a friend on the telephone. Touch is the basis of much of our sensory experiences and the development of consciousness. Think of a baby, it spends a great deal of time exploring the world by means of touch, as well as by taste! Even as adults, with physical objects we can only learn so much by vision, then to really know them we have to touch them – much to the chagrin of the sculpture gallery's attendants!

Practice: We can extend our conscious experience of the body from the feet to the legs. Think for a moment about standing. When we stand our feet are being supported by the floor. I hope that this is obvious and non controversial. We can then go on with the earlier exercise, not just 'thinking about it' but of actively *becoming conscious of this reality*.

These are quite different kinds of activity. When we 'think about' something we separate ourselves from it, we can cut ourselves off from what we are thinking about, we are literally in our heads. On the other hand when we are conscious of a reality, we are able, in Alexander's words 'to be sensorially aware'. We are committed to the here and now not the then and there of thinking about.

I hope that you have already experienced some interesting changes in your perceptions and that physical changes have actually occurred. If you have not had any real experience of increased sensitivity and the reality of the support under your feet, do not despair. In our rather unphysical, technological civilization, many people need time and help for this. However, whatever your experience, be encouraged by the realization that when you are standing, the statement 'my feet are being supported by the floor' *must* be true. It is an ordinary physical fact. Further, the statement 'my lower legs

119

are being supported by my feet' must also be true under
these conditions.

We can continue this process through the rest of the
body to the head, following the route of the supporting
reflexes to the point where the head returns to a free
balance on the neck as the neck muscles spontaneously
release. [6] Being conscious of their action, perhaps with
the aid of touch, helps us in a number of important
ways. Let's review them at this point, drawing together
research and experience.

Bringing it all together

This is part of the process of calibrating our subjective
experiences against objective reality. It is also a part of
the answer to those who claim that the Alexander
Technique is just subjective. Practised well it is not.
Having placed myself under the scrutiny of objective,
verifiable scientific equipment under controlled
laboratory conditions, I can verify it. These tests did more
than verify the Alexander Technique, they also allowed
me to make fuller and finer calibrations to my subjective
experiences and so improve the accuracy of my feelings.
This ability to check my feelings allowed an increase in
the effectiveness of the methods used, further increasing
the accuracy of the feelings and the results on the body.

Becoming conscious of the reality of the support
system and the quality of freedom its natural working
allows our bodies, gives us an experience from the inside
of ourselves – of the here and now. We have reviewed all
the reasons for this to be true from scientific research.
Now we move to the phase of really putting our trust in
it. Alexander found this over 100 years ago. For him it
was much tougher because he only had his own
experiences to go on and the reasoning he applied to
them. Now we have much more to back us up, and yet,
this is a lonely moment . . . we can only do it for ourselves
in the end.

You stand and let yourself be conscious of *your* feet on
the floor, being supported by it, and of the support *your*

feet in turn are giving to *your* legs. It is the result of your conscious decision taken in the face of a lifetime of neglecting such realities, in a culture that in part even denies their existence, let alone their usefulness. These habits, part cultural, part personal are much of what has formed us; in one sense they are us. At this point it might be worth you looking again at pages 33 and 34 for a brief sketch of some of the historical causes of misuse of the body. Now, however, we are dealing with the nuts and bolts of what we are going to do about it and the practical difficulties we face.

This process of consciously choosing to attend to these realities stops our subconscious patterns of interference with the support system. No matter how difficult the practice of this is, it remains a verifiable fact. With the help of a friend or a suitably trained teacher – and patience – the reality of these reflexes and their effects on the body as a whole are there to be experienced. Once begun, our interest makes possible being more sensitive and so being able to receive more information. This information stimulates more interest, leading to more sensitivity, and thus our being able to learn yet more – which stimulates more interest and so on in a naturally reinforcing cycle. The result is a spontaneous release of the body from held habits which often have caused pain and prevented the full expression of our potential.

Real spontaneity
That conscious choosing causes real spontaneity, as well as solving problems, is a surprising concept. Until we realize that, what we normally think of as spontaneous is in reality unthinking habit. Using the ideas of quantum theory, habit is the brain working within the high probability grooves of business as usual. On the other hand being truly in the here and now, by taking time to be more conscious of our bodies, takes us out of this cul de sac to what is more really new and spontaneous. Alternatively, expressing habit in terms of control theory, it is closer to the regularity of a damaged control system

than the controlled unpredictability of a well-functioning, complex, natural one.

Notes

1. For those surprised by this sequence, see Stevens C and Hesse A 'The Primary Control: a new look at Alexander's discovery' *STAT News* September 1995
2. Stevens C (1995) *Yoga*, 3rd Edition (Know the Game series), A&C Black, London
3. Alexander FM (1972) 'Teaching Quotations', *The Alexander Journal*, No.7: p.44. STAT Books, London.
4. Sherrington CH (1947) *The Integrative Action of the Nervous System*, p.232, Cambridge University Press
5. Stevens C (1995) *Towards a Physiology of the Alexander Technique*, STAT Books
6. For a detailed description of this phase of the work and those which follow it see Stevens C and Kevan N 'New directions in the Alexander Technique', in press.

USEFUL ADDRESSES

Further information and a list of qualified teachers of the Alexander Technique can be obtained from the following addresses. Please enclose a large stamped addressed envelope with your enquiry.

UNITED KINGDOM

Society of Teachers of the Alexander Technique (STAT)
20 London House
266 Fulham Road
London SW10 9EL
Tel: 0171 351 0828
Fax: 0171 352 1556

Chris Stevens   or   c/o Professor N. Kevan
45 Penns Court   Georg-Baur-Ring 14
Steyning   D-45133 Essen
West Sussex BN44 3BF   Germany
                                   Tel: 49 201 413504
                                   Fax: 49 201 424898

CANADA

Canadian Society of Teachers of the Alexander Technique (CANSTAT)
460 Palmerston Boulevard
Toronto
Ontario
P7A 4A2

AUSTRALIA

Australian Society of Teachers of the Alexander Technique (AUSTAT)
PO Box 529
Milsons Point
Sydney 2061
New South Wales

FURTHER READING

The Alexander Principle, Dr Wilfred Barlow
(Gollancz, 1973)

More Talk of Alexander, Dr Wilfred Barlow
(Gollancz, 1978)

The Use of the Self, F M Alexander (latest edition,
Gollancz, 1986)

The Constructive Conscious Control of the Individual,
F M Alexander (latest edition, Centerline Press,
1986)

The Man Who Mistook his Wife for a Hat, Oliver Sacks
(Paladin, 1986)

'Form and Function of the Erect Human Spine' in
Orthopaedics and Related Research, volume 25, pages
55-63. E Asmussen and K Klausen (1963)

'Alignment of the Human Body in Standing' in the
European Journal of Applied Physiology, pages
109-115, A M Woodhull et al (1985)

'Lumbar disc pressure and myoelectric back muscle
activity during sitting', *Scandinavian Journal of
Rehabilitation Medicine*, volume 6, pages 104-114,
B J Andersson et al (1974)

The Cause of Lumbar Back Pain, John Gorman
(John Gorman, 1984)

Yoga in the 'Know the Game' series, Chris Stevens
(A & C Black, 1985)

The Endeavour of Jean Fernel, Sir Charles Sherrington
  (Cambridge University Press, 1946)

Body Awareness in Action, Professor F P Jones
  (latest edition, Schocken, 1979)

Body Learning, Michael Gelb (Aurum Press, 1981)

*Medical and Physiological Aspects of the Alexander
  Technique*, Chris Stevens (editor) (Alexander
  Research Press, 1988)

Experimental Studies in the FM Alexander Technique,
  Chris Stevens (Alexander Research Press, 1992)

OTHER BOOKS & ARTICLES
By Chris Stevens

*The Alexander Technique: Medical and Physiological
  Aspects*. Conference Proceedings, latest edition, 1994.

'The influence of initial posture on movement', *European
  Journal of Applied Physiology*. Research Paper, 1989.

*Scientific Research and its Role in Teaching the Alexander
  Technique*. Alexander Memorial Lecture, 1990.

Research into the effects of the Alexander Technique.
  Summarised results of scientific studies, 1994.

Towards a Physiology of the Alexander Technique.
  An overview of the mechanisms underlying the
  Technique drawn from the author's studies, 1995.

Most of these publications are available from STAT
Books, 20 London House, 266 Fulham Road, London
SW10 9EL. Tel. 0171 351 0828. Fax. 0171 352 1556.

INDEX